When a young child first produces speech in sentences it is the end product of an exciting process of communication and development of understanding that begins from the moment of birth. The fascinating process of how babies learn to communicate with the world around them is attractively and accessibly presented in this delightful, original and thoughtful book.

Máire Messenger Davies is a journalist of many years' experience and was a previous deputy editor of *Mother & Baby* magazine. She is currently a free-lance adviser and contributor to *Parents* magazine, while also researching her PhD thesis on the effects of television on learning. She is author of *The Breastfeeding Book* (Century).

Both Eva Lloyd and Andreas Scheffler are psychology graduates. Eva Lloyd is a researcher at the Thomas Coram Research Unit, London. Andreas Scheffler is currently employed by Haringey Health Authority, and has a special interest in the development and application of cognitive psychology.

BABY LANGUAGE

MÁIRE MESSENGER DAVIES, EVA LLOYD and ANDREAS SCHEFFLER

Photographs by John Campbell

London
UNWIN PAPERBACKS
Boston Sydney Wellington

First published by Unwin Paperbacks 1987

This book is copyright under the Berne Convention.
No reproduction without permission. All rights reserved.

UNWIN® PAPERBACKS
A Division of Unwin Hyman Ltd
40 Museum Street, London WC1A 1LU, UK

Unwin Paperbacks
A Division of Unwin Hyman Ltd
Park Lane, Hemel Hempstead, Herts HP2 4TE, UK

Allen & Unwin Australia Pty Ltd
8 Napier Street, North Sydney, NSW 2060, Australia

Unwin Paperbacks with the
Port Nicholson Press
PO Box 11–838 Wellington, New Zealand

Copyright © Máire Messenger Davies,
Eva Lloyd and Andreas Scheffler 1987

© Photographs by John Campbell

British Library Cataloguing in Publication Data

Davies, Máire Messenger
  Baby language.
1. Children—Language   2. Infants
I. Title   II. Scheffler, Andreas
III. Lloyd, Eva
401'.9   LB1139.L3
ISBN 0–04–649041–8

Set in 11 on 13 point Souvenir by Bedford Typesetters Limited, Bedford,
and printed in Great Britain by The Bath Press, Avon

Contents

Foreword   7

1. What is Language?   9
2. What is a Baby?   23
3. Crying   37
4. Body Language   53
5. The First Non-Crying Sounds   63
6. First Words   73
7. Two Words and Beyond   85
8. The Wider World of Language   94
9. Bilingual Babies   111
10. Is Language Developing Normally?   123

Useful Addresses   131

Booklist   132

References   133

Index   139

Foreword

This book is about the developments which take place in your baby which enable him or her to learn to speak and understand; it starts with the newborn baby and ends at around the age of two and a half when a child has started to produce sentences. We hope to show that producing sentences is only the end product of an exciting process of communication, play and 'trial and error' which goes on in the early months and years, before 'proper' speech emerges.

It cannot be said often enough that all babies are different, as are all parents. We have given very rough indications of when particular stages in language development occur, because this is helpful but it does not mean that *every baby* should be reaching these stages at precisely this age. There is *very wide variation* in the rate at which a child learns the language, and in the amount of language that he or she uses. In the last chapter there are some guidelines which may help to give you an idea of whether you should be worried about your child's language development, but we hope that, in general, this is a reassuring book that expresses the interest and excitement of language learning.

Another proviso is that we have talked mainly about English. Also many of the studies we have referred to are based on small groups of children, and you may very well find that *your* child is doing something different from what the research suggests is 'normal'. This is no cause for concern and is another reassuring example of the great flexibility and creativity of the skills of language learning.

We have addressed 'you' the reader, assuming that 'you' are probably the baby's mother or mother-figure. This is only for convenience; we hope that 'you' are just as likely to be the baby's father or childminder or nurse, or any other person who is interested in babies – or, indeed, in language. We have referred to the baby as 'he' in some chapters and 'she' in others, so that both sexes are acknowledged.

We have referred to the children in our own families – Thomas, Hannah, Huw, Elinor, Kate, Owen, Alastair, James and Nicolas – in giving examples of children's language development. We are also grateful to the many other children and parents who have provided examples for this book.

We would like to thank Dr Anne Woollett of the North East London Polytechnic Psychology Department, Eveline de Jong and Pam Stevenson for their help and advice in preparing the book. We would also like to thank all the families who gave their time to be photographed for the book.

Máire Messenger Davies
Eva Lloyd
Andreas Scheffler

1

What is Language?

> Kate (aged four) on seeing a picture of the Loch Ness Monster in a children's book: 'That monster is only imaginary, isn't it, mummy?'

By the time a child is four years old, long before he is physically, socially or emotionally mature, he has mastered all the basic adult language skills. Like Kate, a four-year-old can use complex grammar, such as a question with an added tag ('isn't it?'). He can use difficult words, referring to abstract concepts ('imaginary') and his speech will reflect a surprisingly wide knowledge of the outside world and the controversies in it ('the Loch Ness monster'; '*only* imaginary').

You may think that the time, usually during the second year, when a toddler starts combining two or more words is the point at which 'proper' speech miraculously emerges. 'He's started to talk,' says grandma approvingly. Yet, as soon as they are born, we interpret the noises our babies make as if they are meaningful, and we talk and coo to them as if they understand us. Parents instinctively treat their babies as partners in conversation.

Speech is universally seen as one of the most important and unique characteristics of human beings. The first word, a milestone in your baby's development, is eagerly awaited. It is hardly surprising that the sounds of the first 'real' words used by Japanese babies are identical to those used by English-speaking babies! Universal babbling sounds, made by babies all over the world, such as 'papa', 'dada', 'mama', 'baba' and 'nana' have been taken by parents and families everywhere as being directed at them personally. The baby, who had not quite intended these sounds like that, is naturally encouraged by the enthusiasm he has generated in his parents – and the mutually-exciting process of speech development is on its way. But long before the emergence of these first words, the baby was already 'talking' to his parents.

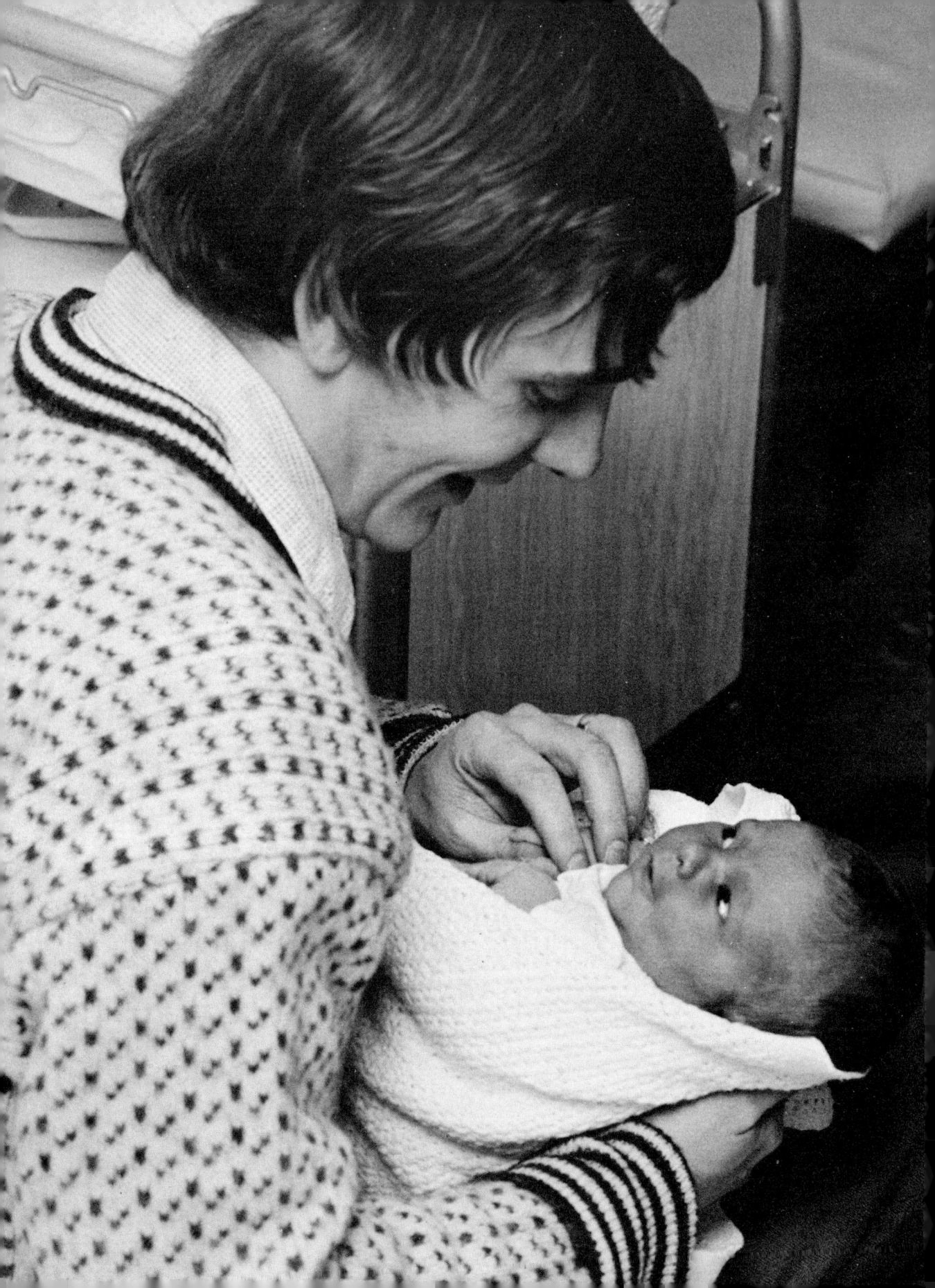

From the start parent and baby are partners in conversation.

In this book we hope to show you how language learning begins at birth and how you and your baby are equal partners in this venture. We hope to point out ways in which all the developmental steps taken by your baby can be seen as aids in your child's transition from pre-verbal communication to speech. Hopefully, the following chapters will reassure you that your baby's natural inclination to talk is so strong that you need not worry unduly about the best way to teach him actively to speak, or to speak correctly.

All the experts on language acquisition agree about the fact that parents make it possible for children to develop language by acting naturally. By introducing your baby to the fascinating world around you, by sharing his interests and letting him share your enjoyment of everyday things, including conversation, you are giving him an optimal start as a talker. *How* parents speak is not nearly so important as whether they talk to their babies at all: several studies have shown that mothers who talk to their babies a lot have children with larger vocabularies at eighteen months, although other children do catch up eventually.[1]

The early signs of language development often prompt parents to ask some wider questions about the how and why of language. The first attempts at speaking made by a small child make us much more acutely aware of the fascination and mystique of words.

What is language?

Speaking and language are not the same thing. (For instance, some deaf people can understand written language and can communicate in visual signs, although they cannot talk.) But speaking is the main way in which human beings communicate through language, and a baby learning to speak is the clearest sign that he is beginning to use language effectively. So we will start with speech.

Speech has been described as 'an extremely efficient use of spent air'. Human beings are equipped with vocal chords and a mouth capable of modulating the air used in breathing to produce an extensive range of distinct sounds. Further, their hearing organs are able to make fine distinctions between just those kinds of sounds. Babies as young as one month appear to be capable of discriminating between speech sounds such as 'p' and 'b'.[2] We do not know at exactly what point in evolution the human species came to use this endowment for speech, although it must have been relatively recent in human history. There is evidence that Neanderthal man did not possess this capacity for speech, whereas Cro-Magnon man probably did. Both lived around 35,000 years ago.

We do know that in *every* one of the thousands of languages spoken today, a limited number of sound combinations – the *words* of that language – are structured into larger units, such as sentences, according to a limited number of combination-rules – the *grammar* of that language. The way the sounds are combined to form words is also subject to rules in each language. Language 'families' exist, made up of languages whose sound-systems and grammars are related, but the differences between these families are considerable. English is part of the Germanic branch of the Indo-European languages, as are Dutch, Icelandic, Danish and German.

It is generally accepted that there must be a common structure underlying all languages, hard though it is to define, since they can all ultimately be translated into each other and they all fulfil the same function. This common structure is sometimes called a universal grammar. If you are in a bi-lingual family, you might find it interesting to think about ways in which your two (or more) languages are similar and ways in which they differ. There is more information about bi-lingual babies in Chapter 9.

The words and grammar of their language allow speakers to be endlessly creative in the combinations they make, so that almost every sentence ever spoken is new. Of course we also use a stock of greetings, traditional sayings and other ritual phrases ('Never mind', 'I told you so' and so on). A child learning to speak becomes creative in this sense as soon as he starts combining two or more words.

In speaking, we vary the tone of our voice according to the context and situation, as when asking questions; the questioning tone is used by children who are still only using single words. Our voice also varies according to our mood. In English, a loud voice is often an angry voice and at two months this emotional tone of voice will make babies cry. We also accompany our words with gestures, of which pointing is one of the first to emerge, and our 'body language' often betrays the true meaning of our words. Have you noticed how a toddler squirms when you catch him out at a fib?

There is very little relationship between the *sounds* of words and the things they refer to (referents); this is why language is called a symbolic system of communication. The number of words in any language which mimic the sound of their referent, such as animal noises ('moo', 'woof') is extremely small. Mostly, words do not sound anything like their meaning and the same sound can mean quite different things in different languages ('oui' in French and 'wee' in English, for example). Language enables us to talk to fellow speakers about common and new experiences in the past, the present and the future, about places seen and

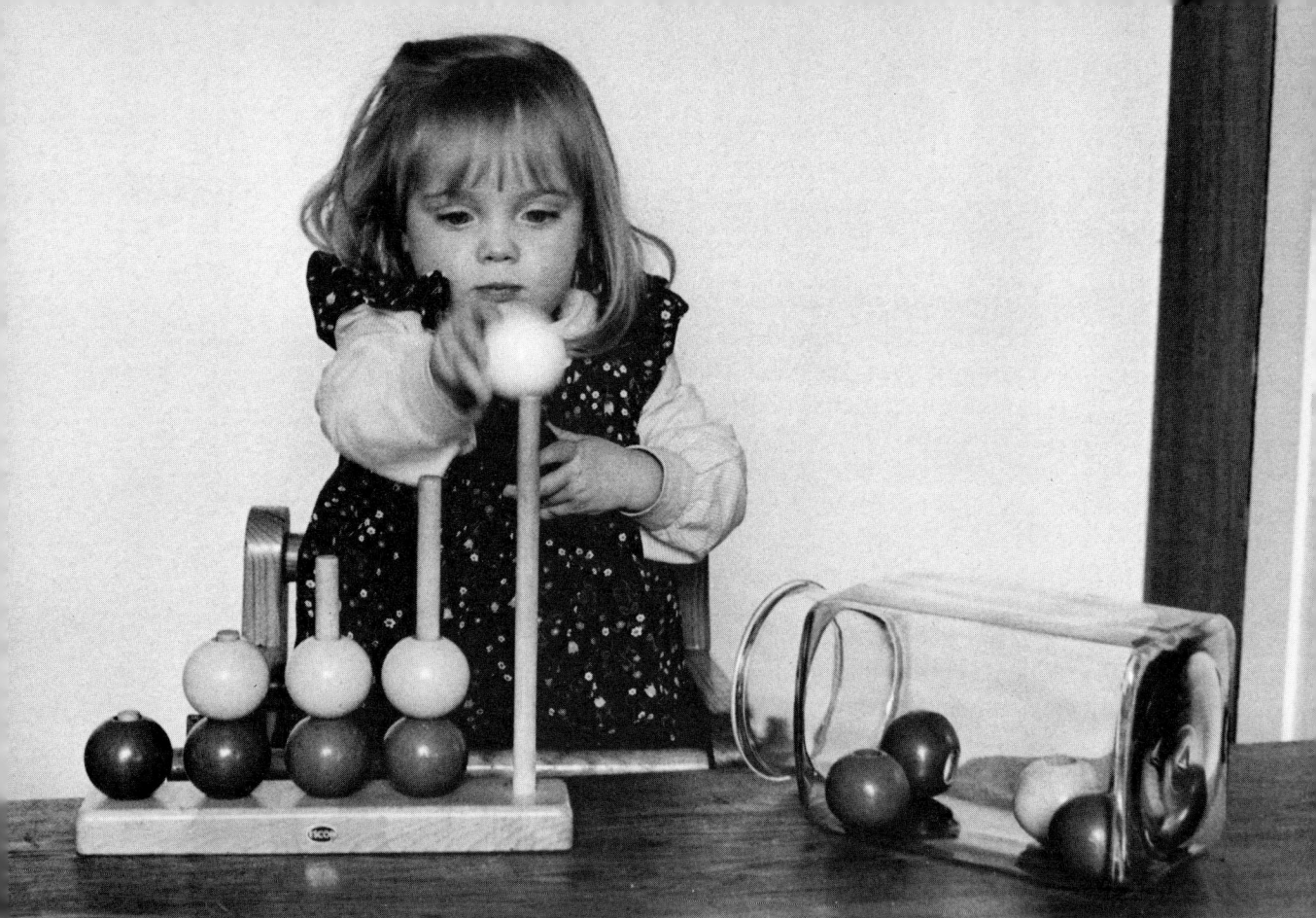

Learning to categorise – blue things, hard things, round things.

unseen and about real and imaginary things. It is one of our greatest assets in learning because it allows us to acquire knowledge about objects, concepts, events and feelings, without the immediate need for direct experience.

Language makes learning about the world easier because we can *label* all its different aspects that are relevant to our lives. Learning names for colours, shapes and sizes, for instance, helps a child to *categorise* objects (an important intellectual skill) in terms of shared features: blue things, round things, big things. Ultimately, this helps the child to learn to identify the underlying concepts: blue, red, orange are all colours; round, square, triangular are all shapes; big, small, wide, narrow, fat, thin are all ways of describing something's size.

Language is dynamic in adapting to our changing environment: we coin new words for new objects and experiences and drop the ones that no longer apply, or we change their meanings. The rules of grammar also change over time; in English, for instance, we no longer inflect verbs – 'thou comest', 'he goeth', and so on. A modern one-year-old may make the acquaintance of a home computer before setting eyes on a typewriter. Lottie happily labelled her 'first' typewriter with 'puter'!

We see the extent to which language makes fast and efficient learning possible when we look at the achievements of a four-year-old. (By four, children have mastered all the basic rules of their language.)

The language of a four-year-old

We all know that the average baby does not exist, but what follows is generally true of four-year-olds who live in a family or good institution. The four-year-old's vocabulary encompasses all kinds of words: verbs, nouns, prepositions and grown-up sounding ones like 'actually', with which many sophisticated fours preface their remarks. Nevertheless, the finer shades of meaning of the approximately 1550 words they now use are still to become apparent to them and they will be puzzled by irony or sarcasm.

'What does so and so mean?' has become a favourite question as the four-year-old has had so much practice with the sounds of his language that he easily retains words that he does not understand. He makes far fewer errors in pronunciation than a year ago and may regard trying to imitate difficult words you say as a challenge.

Four-year-olds are very sensitive to qualities such as rhyme and will make up little verses themselves. They will also find hackneyed expressions such as 'easy as pie' amusing, since these expressions have not yet lost their freshness for them. Hearing herself say 'I do not know' in answer to a question, Molly remembered to add: 'Said the great bell of Bow'.

At four, a child is well aware of the existence of grammatical rules, so much so that he finds exceptions hard to cope with. Whereas he might have used 'said', 'went' and 'taken' in imitation of you a year ago, he will now experiment with 'sayed' and 'goed' and 'tooken' which conform to the patterns he has identified for forming the past tense of verbs.

He pays close attention to word order to help him work out who does what to whom in the sentences you use to him. One of his current 'rules' tells him that the first noun in any sentence refers to the actor or 'doer'. Therefore he neither understands nor uses a passive construction like 'Teddy is kissed by the dolly'. He will only understand 'The dolly kisses Teddy', and you can test him on this by asking him to act out sentences like these with his toys. The chances are that whoever is mentioned first in the sentence, Teddy or dolly, will be the one doing the kissing. In fact, adults rarely use passives in talking to pre-school children, although there can be some specific experiences where they can be meaningful. On hearing of a visit to the hairdresser or the hospital, a four-year-old may ask: 'What did you have done to you?'

Generally, the four-year-old's sentences are complex and full of 'ifs' and 'becauses'. However, he can be bemused by a sentence such as 'Before Johnny went to bed he brushed his teeth' and even has trouble imitating it after you. For him, it is first things first: he expects the order in which events are described to follow the real-life order of events. So 'Johnny brushed his teeth before he went to bed' presents no problems.

Having already developed into a well-rounded social being, the four-year-old is keen to use ritual phrases: 'Did I hear anyone say "bless you"?' Kate inquired huffily when her sneeze in company was met by silence all round. Although the child's perspective on time is different from yours, he can discuss his past and his future with you and can distinguish between real and imaginary in his everyday experience. He may not be able to do this with television programmes, however, in which a drama can seem as real as a documentary and in which the news can seem like a cops and robbers story. You can usefully help him to sort out the different techniques (such as commentators, presenters, interviews, captions) which distinguish 'real-life' material on TV from fictional material (which will have background music, dialogue, ritualised actions). Understanding these things will be a valuable protection against the kinds of 'harmful' influences of television that so many parents worry about.

When rising-fives start infant school they are introduced to writing – that valuable system for making communication permanent and helping the spread of information. A four-year-old will hopefully have had several years' experience of reading, at least in the form of being read to. He may arrive at school knowing his alphabet, or some of it. In our multi-cultural society, he will find out that some children at his school speak a different language at home. This adds yet another dimension to his already sophisticated knowledge about the world, as well as about language.

Learning different languages

Despite the existence of so many different languages, there is ample evidence that all children of all nations pass through similar stages in language learning, although individuals differ in the ages at which they progress from one stage to the next – as you may have noticed if you have more than one child. Cooing and babbling are universal; the more language the baby hears, the more he will coo and babble. In some cultures, parents direct little 'babytalk' at cooing and babbling babies, but older brothers and sisters do. This subject is covered in more detail in Chapter 5.

Children everywhere put all they want to say into single words before they express relationships between objects and events in two-word statements. At around the same age, the English child may say 'brick fall', the Samoan one 'fall doll' ('p'u pepe') and the Finnish child 'Seppo fall' ('Seppo putoo').[3]

An American linguist, Dan Slobin, has investigated the *order* in which certain language functions emerge in different languages.[4] The here-and-now is the subject of conversations everywhere when children first use single words. This similarity in everyday topics (food, clothes, toys, familiar people) remains as the child progresses to the next more complex phase; children talk about their direct experiences, they describe, ask, refuse, deny. But if a grammatical rule is unusually complex in a particular language, the correct expression takes longer to learn for children speaking that language than for other children. An instance of such complexity is the use of the possessive in English. At first a small child will say 'Katie shoe'; then she will learn the correct 'Katie's shoe'. But the use of the word 'of', as in 'the shoe of Katie' will present problems for some time to come.

The idea of plurality – that something can be more than one – occurs to children everywhere at around the age of two and they find ways of expressing this understanding. Yet, while English-speaking children have mastered the general rule of plural-formation (add 's' or 'es') and a large number of exceptions to it (mice, sheep, knives) by the time they are six, Egyptian children do not use all the grammatically correct forms in Egyptian Arabic until they are teenagers, as these are much more complex.[5]

Dan Slobin gives a striking example of this process operating in two children who were bilingual in Hungarian and Serbo-Croat.[6] By two years and six months they could talk about putting things *on* tables and *in* boxes, but the correct grammatical form for expressing 'in' and 'on' was acquired in Hungarian almost six months before the equivalent construction in Serbo-Croat, as the Hungarian form was easier.

All children appear to have a way of paying attention to the *ends* of words rather than to their beginnings. Thus, grammatical information attached to the end of the word or phrase is more easily learned and produced than if it is given before the word. The article 'the' in English, which always comes before the noun, is learned later than its equivalent form in Rumanian, which is attached to the end of the noun. (In Rumanian, 'wolf' is 'lup' and 'the wolf' is 'lupul'.)

Intellectual development determines the order in which certain grammatical constructions are learned, irrespective of whether they are easy or difficult. In Russian, for instance, expressing an 'if' or hypothetical idea is easier than in English. But English children start using constructions like 'If it is sunny, we'll go to the park tomorrow' at the same age as Russian children; when they are

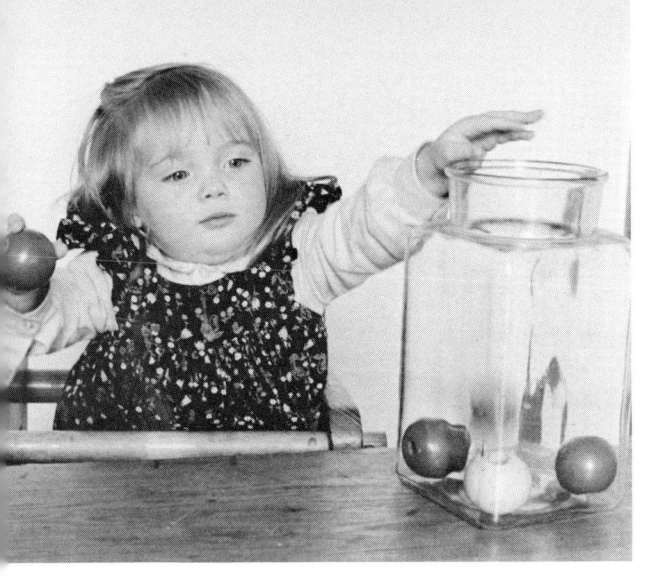
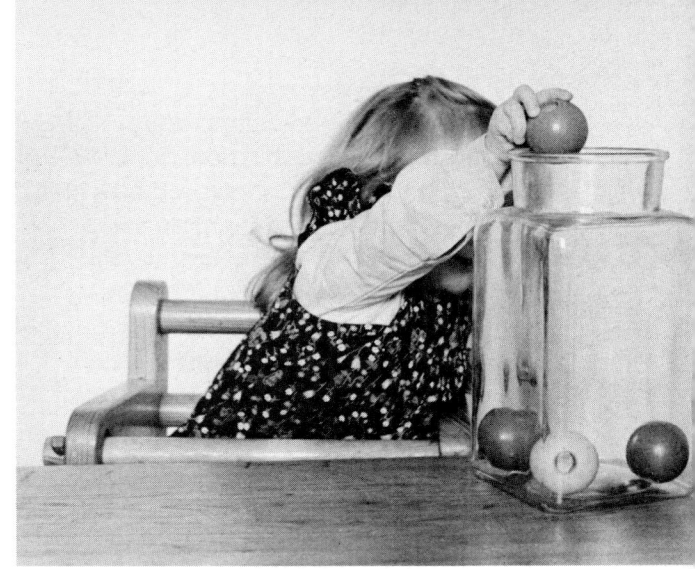
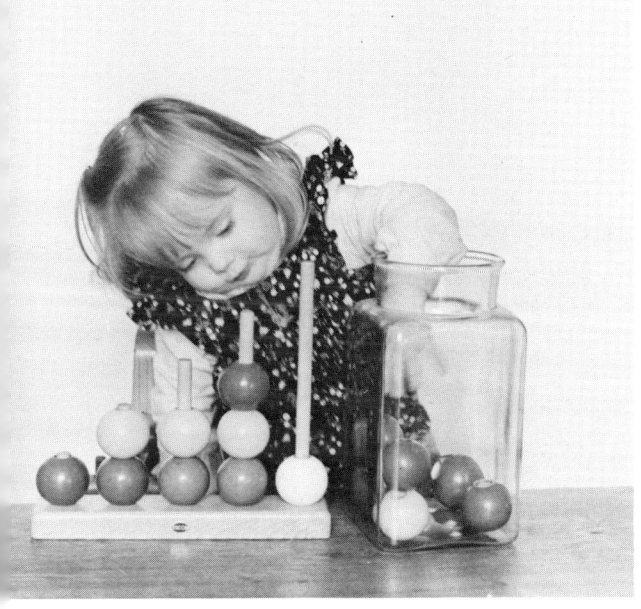
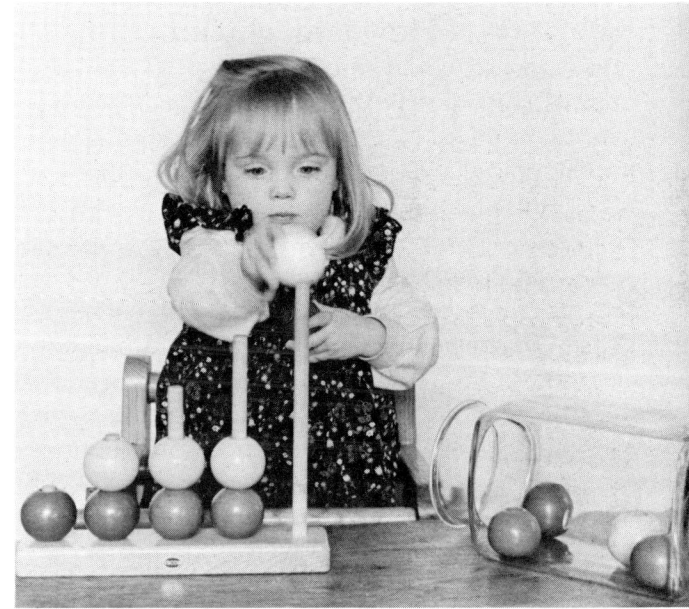
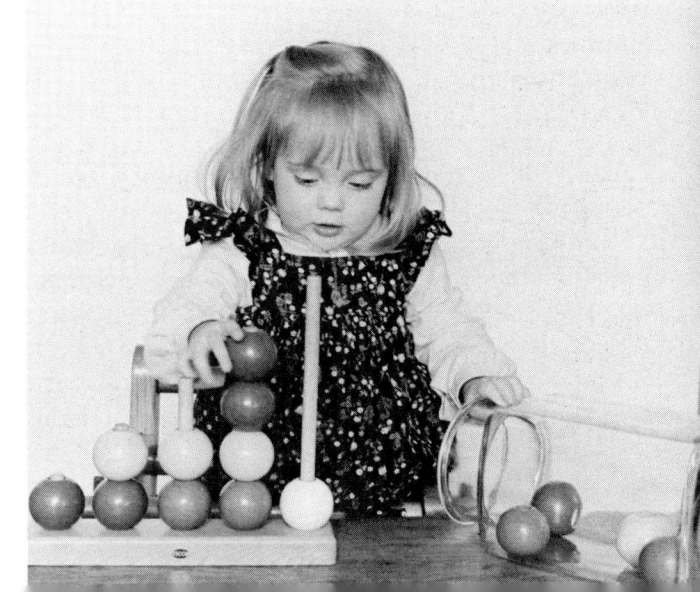

Consequences – 'If I put the ball in here,.... then tip the jar.... then I can get the red one for my tower'.

intellectually capable of understanding 'if... then' they can also manage the more difficult verbal construction. 'Put the ball in the cup' is a request universally understood by a child of around two because it follows his natural inclination to do so. But 'put the cup over the ball' may get no response because, from his point of view, there is not much point in such an action.

It appears that the strategies many children apply to language learning also serve the purpose of helping them to make sense of the world in which this language is used. Although they receive a lot of help and encouragement from you and from other people, children seem to have their own very effective ways of teaching themselves how to use language. Many researchers have tried to answer the question every parent is bound to ask: how does the child manage to learn to speak in such a short time?

How and why language?

Some people would argue that the child learns by imitation of his parents. But only a little reflection is necessary to see that imitation cannot be the whole answer. Naturally, imitation is responsible for extending vocabulary and for the fact that the child speaks in his parents' language and has the same accent they have. But the child uses grammatical rules creatively when combining single words into longer utterances. Children do not hear their parents say 'Katie shoe' or 'goed' or 'mans', yet you have almost certainly heard your own child or other children make logical 'mistakes' like this.

In the early stages of speech development, the child is actually incapable of imitating certain sound combinations correctly, even though he can perceive them. The linguist Neil Smith has given many amusing examples of his three-year-old son's irritation at being corrected:

Father: Say 'jump'.
Child: Dup.
Father: No, 'jump'.
Child: Dup.
Father: No, 'jummp'.
Child: Only Daddy can say dup.[7]

Neil Smith's little boy was right: he knew what the word should *sound* like, that is, how his father pronounced it. But he knew that he could not manage it himself. There are limitations on what constructions and pronunciations can be imitated by a child at any one stage. At the two word stage, imitation of longer sentences spoken by adults is reduced by the child to two words – normally the main topic words. 'Mummy is making a drink' becomes 'mummy drink'. Children even find it difficult to imitate their own sentences, particularly more complex ones that are longer than their usual statements for the stage they are at. For instance, a two-year-old may come up with an 'if' sentence – not normally in regular use until the fourth year: 'If you're not good, we won't have any sweets' he may admonish his teddy. If you ask him to repeat this, it is likely that he will find it quite impossible.

Although children cannot imitate their own more sophisticated sayings, it is likely that they pick up such sayings by imitation in the first place. Owen (twenty-one months) had not used very many words at all when he heard his sister say 'I can hear Mizzy meowing'. 'So can I', announced Owen. Kate and her father looked around for an undetected fourth speaker, as they could hardly believe these sophisticated words had passed Owen's lips.

Imitation or inborn?

Many prominent researchers used to argue that imitation was the whole explanation for language learning. The American psychologist, B. F. Skinner, called language 'verbal behaviour' – and he argued that, like other forms of behaviour, language developed as a response to prompting from the parents.[8] According to this theory, parents reward sounds which seem like words with food and attention – so the baby learns to repeat them. Incorrect or meaningless noises are supposed to be ignored and so the child learns not to use them. The child learns to produce only those imitations of his parents' speech that appear to have the desired consequences of food or attention.

It is hard to believe that psychologists who developed such theories ever put them to the test. Parents know only too well that babies get their needs met so effectively merely by crying, that it is a miracle they bother to learn adult language at all! As we shall see in later chapters, *all* noises made by babies, no matter how apparently meaningless, are interpreted by parents as having meaning and draw attention to the baby very effectively. When the first words appear, parents respond to content rather than form; it is not 'correctness' that they are concerned about, but meaning. When Elinor (twenty-one months) laboriously put together her first sentence: 'Where's mama cuppatea?', she was hugged by everybody (and, of course, answered – 'It's on the table'.) No one bothered to correct her grammar; everyone was too delighted with her achievement.

At three years or so, parents explicitly correct forms like 'goed' and 'tooths' but word-order mistakes like 'What it is?' are hardly noticed. Systematic experiments have confirmed that efforts to turn a child's remarks into grammatically correct versions have no effect on the rate at which these correct versions are acquired.[9] The *interest* you show in what your child is trying to say appears to offer all the encouragement necessary.

Skinner's imitation theory was heavily criticised by the American linguist, Noam Chomsky, whose own grammatical theory became very popular in the 'sixties.[10] According to Chomsky, we are endowed by nature with a Language Acquisition Device, a set of universal grammatical rules enabling us to learn the particular grammar of our own language from the complex and often imperfect speech of our parents.[11] Without this inborn system it would take us more than a life-time to acquire our native language by imitation and reward alone. The controversy between these two points of view is another example of the 'nature or nurture' argument. Are newborn children innately equipped with the intelligence for learning different skills or are they, as the philosopher John Locke put it, blank sheets of paper on which the environment writes its lessons?

You probably have your own idea as to the answer to this question, particularly if you already have a baby or two. As far as language is concerned, it is now generally accepted that the baby is born with a predisposition to acquire speech (some of the fascinating evidence for this is given in Chapter 2) but not all of Chomsky's arguments can be demonstrated. For instance, he argued that simple grammatical forms are learned before more complex ones. According to this view, negative forms such as 'can't', 'won't' and 'don't' should be learned later than the positive forms 'can', 'will' and 'do', because negatives are more complex. In fact, 'can't', 'won't' and 'don't' *do* come before 'can', 'will' and 'do' in children's early speech – which says a great deal about the personality of the average toddler![12]

Chomsky also described adults' speech to children as defective, but there is ample evidence that parents use a special kind of simple and highly grammatical speech to their children, which is geared to their level of understanding.[13] Tone of voice is also important in creating meaning; even at the one word stage, children formulate questions by using a rising intonation 'daddy?' (Where's daddy gone?) and their words are interpreted by their parents as meaning different things in different situations. If parents misunderstand, they manage to make it clear from their tone whether they want their child to repeat his request or observation, or to rephrase it.

It soon became obvious to researchers that speech development cannot be seen as separate from the child's relationships with parents, siblings and other caretakers (discussed again in later chapters); nor can it be separated from the growth of his *understanding*.

If you observe your baby, you will quickly realise that understanding about the world has to come before he can start using

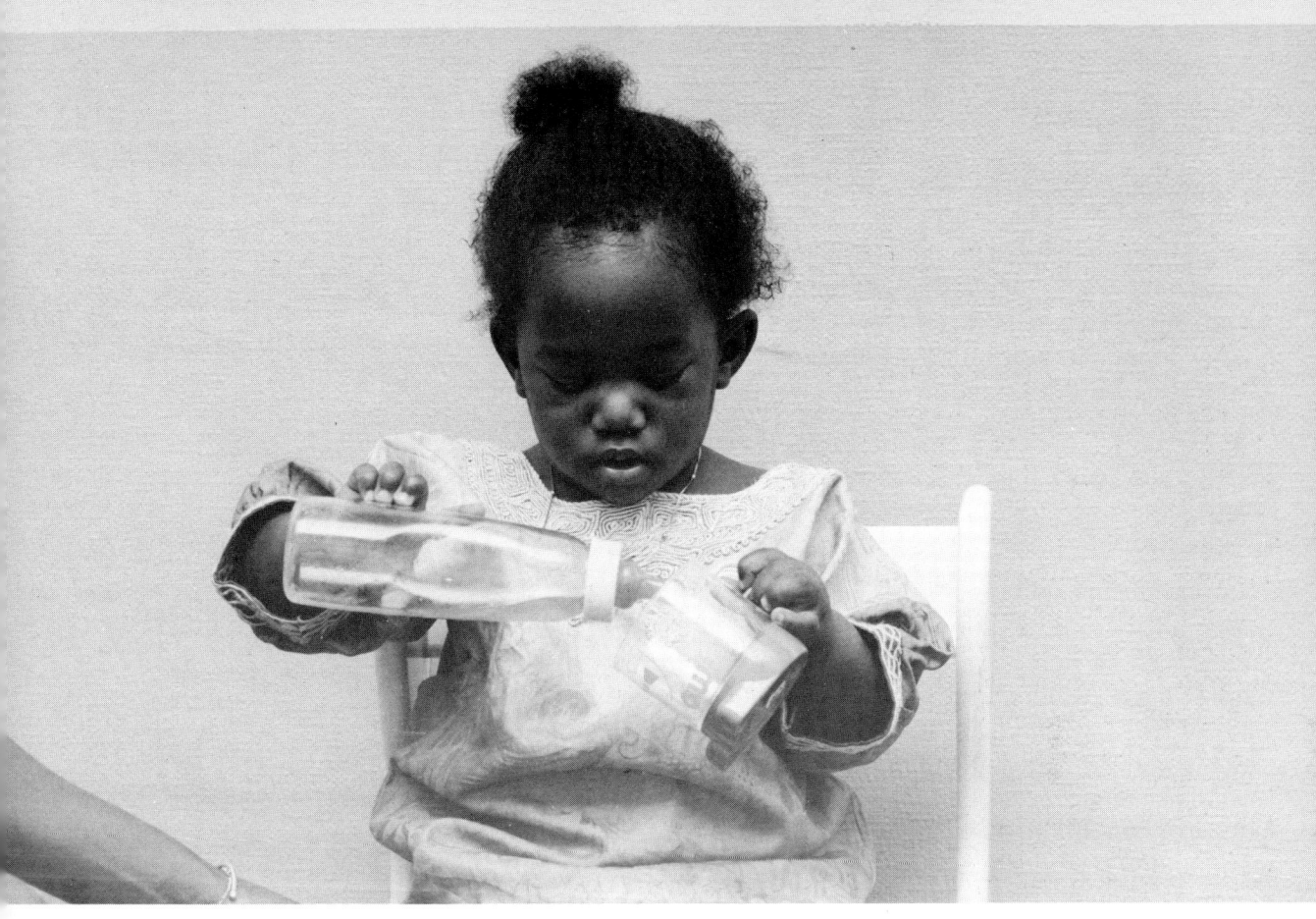

The function of things – a bottle is for pouring.

language properly. For instance, he has to understand that objects, such as plates and toys, have a separate, permanent existence which goes on all the time, even when they are out of sight, before he can give them names and talk about them when they are not there. This intellectual development begins at around four to five months but may not fully mature until the second year. He has to understand the different *functions* of things: a cup is for drinking, a truck is for pushing, a brick is for building, before he can use verbs which describe those functions. In the early months, all objects are for grabbing and eating; it is only towards the end of the first year that the important sense of function develops, and then you will notice it developing very rapidly.

However, language development can show some interesting exceptions to this general rule that the understanding of a concept has to exist before it can be put into words. The researcher, Richard Cromer, has demonstrated that children can understand a concept such as 'fun' quite easily, but not all the constructions in which the word appears.[14] 'The wolf is fun to bite' can be difficult for children to interpret up to the age of nine or so; 'the wolf is keen to bite' is much more straightforward. 'Fun' presents no problems in other contexts.

'Why' questions also appear before children fully understand that 'why' is related to the concept of cause and effect. Most children automatically progress to 'why' after practising for some time with 'what' and 'where'. Jill and Peter de Villiers, who have studied the language of young children extensively, quote a 26-month-old girl who, when she was told: 'That's the garage door' asked 'Why the garage door?' She actually meant 'Where's the garage door?'[15] It took her a long time to identify 'why' questions as requests for explanations; a few months later she was still confusing 'why' with 'where' as the following conversation shows:

Child: 'I can't wash this.'
Adult: 'Why not?'
Child: 'In here.'

In psychological jargon we could say that understanding is a necessary, but not a sufficient condition for the emergence of grammatical speech, just as the presence of a stimulating environment is. If a child were faced with working out all the grammatical rules of his language from the speech input of his parents and siblings and his growing understanding of his surroundings, it would take many more years to develop into a fluent talker than it actually does. So it does seem as if he has a natural gift for learning and using language creatively, which can operate even in adverse conditions such as neglectful families or bad institutions, but will flourish in a loving home.

2

What is a Baby?

Mother in maternity ward (to her baby). 'Alright darling, let's get you dressed. Oh you are a messy girl.'
(To fellow-mother): 'Anyone looking in here would think we were daft, wouldn't they, talking to a tiny baby like that.'

At one time, not so long ago, the newborn baby was seen by many people as a primitive and passive receiver of external stimulation. The baby's brain was viewed as a blank blackboard waiting to be written on and babies' experiences were described as a 'booming, buzzing confusion'. Over the past few years, attitudes and knowledge have changed dramatically. Today, we know that after nine months of development in the uterus the baby has acquired an already formidable repertoire of skills, which will enable her to manipulate her surroundings and to communicate with others in many different ways.

The newborn baby's ability to perceive through her senses and to start interpreting what she perceives is highly organised at birth. She is able to learn with astonishing speed. A baby's learning is actually faster than at any other time in later life.

Development before birth

In order to understand the skills that the newborn baby brings into the world, it is useful to know some of the developments that have taken place during pregnancy. The baby's life, psychologically as well as physically, begins long before birth. By about the thirteenth week, sensitivity to touch has spread to most parts of the foetus. There are also signs of activities in the nerve centres of the still-forming cortex of the brain. Around this stage, the foetus becomes much more active too. By around sixteen weeks, most of the touch reflexes found in the newborn are present, and by around twenty-four weeks all the sensory systems are working, although a lot of development still has to take place.

Some weeks before birth, too, the baby is capable of carrying out quite complicated movements, such as sucking. Babies have been observed to suck their thumbs in the womb. The various component parts of sucking the thumb may occur fairly early in development; they are then gradually assembled into the complex and more complete co-ordinated pattern of behaviour seen after birth.

Pre-natal experiences

As these developments take place during pregnancy, it follows that events during pre-natal life may affect some of the baby's behaviour immediately after birth. The variety of experience during pregnancy and labour may account for some of the individual differences between newborn babies.

For example, if a mother has been under stress during her pregnancy, she may produce more adrenalin than usual. The baby will become used to this higher level, which may stimulate more activity and restlessness antenatally. It may show up after birth in a higher degree of wakefulness, more activity, differences in her sleeping and waking cycle and perhaps some irritability and difficulty in being soothed. Some of these effects may be short-lived, others may be longer lasting, depending, of course, on the subsequent experiences that the baby has.

The experience of birth

Events occurring during labour also account for some of the individual differences in behaviour noted immediately after birth. A long and stressful labour may result in babies having a more unpredictable sleep pattern – they can be more difficult to settle to sleep, and even when they have achieved this, are more likely to wake up frequently. Drugs given in labour can also affect a baby's behaviour.

Pain-relievers and sedatives pass through the mother's bloodstream into the baby's and, after delivery, can still be passed on in breast milk. Adults are normally very efficient in breaking down excess drugs but the new baby is not – and the drugs will remain for a much longer period in her body. In addition, a mild dose for the mother is quite a hefty dose for the baby. The lasting effects of these drugs can make a baby more sleepy and unwilling to feed, less responsive and less able to activate the learning skills already mentioned. These effects usually pass off after a time, but they can make the early stages of establishing good communication with a baby (including feeding her) more difficult. It helps to be aware of these factors so that, if your baby behaves in a way different from what you have been led to expect, you have some possible explanations. You will need to persevere a bit harder with a baby like this – and to be more patient and tolerant.

First meeting

Most mothers who did not have a general anaesthetic at birth, probably remember their first meeting with their baby very vividly. In common with nearly all mothers who have been studied, they said 'Hallo' to her, or will give her some other kind of greeting. From the start, before the umbilical cord has even been cut, a baby is treated as a partner in conversation. Given the chance, mothers usually touch and stroke their babies all over, and comment on their appearance. Any slight abnormality will be noticed, as will similarities to other family members: 'Oh, he's got your father's nose.'

If the baby is not well at birth (or if the mother is not) there may not be the chance to make this first 'conversational' contact. If this happens to you, as soon as you do get the chance, try to behave as if your meeting with the baby *were* just after birth. Talk to her and greet her as if meeting her for the first time. If the mother is not well, the father can provide the baby's first contacts; these days, since most fathers attend the births of their babies, fathers usually meet their children almost as soon as the mothers do. Babies born at home, or in a short-stay hospital unit, will also soon meet other members of the family – brothers and sisters, grandparents, relatives and friends.

So long as they are not frightened and over-stimulated with too much noise and handling, new babies will be responsive to all loving and friendly approaches. It is especially touching to watch a new baby as an older sibling bends over her cot. You will notice that everybody – even children – speaks to the baby in a higher-pitched voice than usual. This is probably because the baby's hearing is better attuned to high sounds at this stage; it is another fascinating example of how adults and babies seem to be 'pre-programmed' to develop communication with each other.

What is the baby like?

After birth the baby will be weighed, measured and medically checked. The average weight for newborn babies is approximately 7 lb (3.2 kg), but, as with children and adults, there will always be variations in weight and size. Boys normally weigh a few ounces more than girls (on average); if the baby is your first, she will probably be lighter than subsequent babies. If both parents are large, the baby is likely to be large; similarly if both are small, the baby will be smaller. However, the size of the mother's pelvis is a more important determinant of size at birth than any genetic factors; genetic factors determine later growth and size.

With regard to body weight, doctors have drawn an arbitrary line at around 5½ lb (2,500 g) and call all babies under this weight low birth weight. Some of these babies have been born pre-

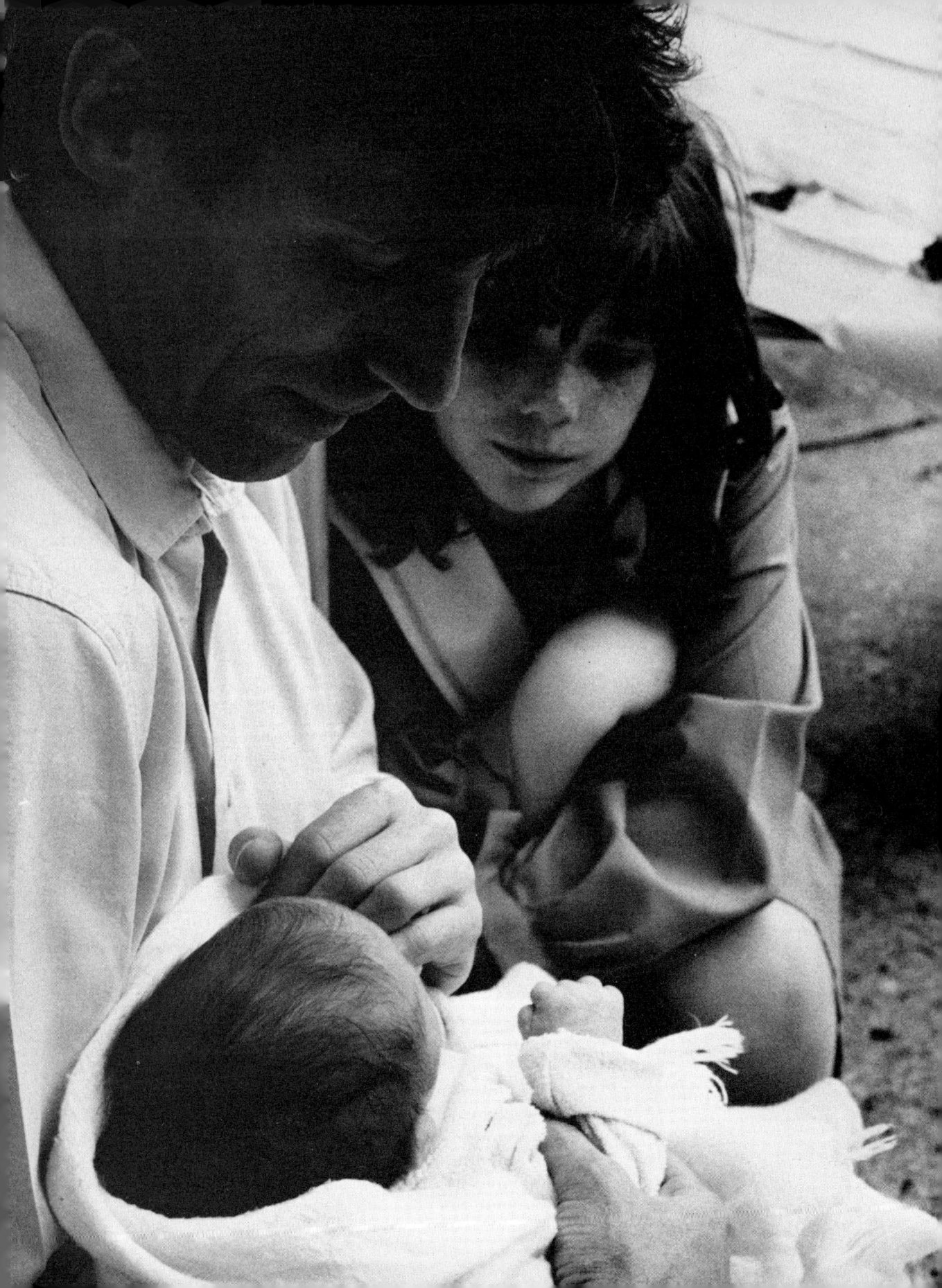

maturely which is why they are small; other babies may be full-term (forty weeks) but still small for their age. Size and weight depend on her growth during pregnancy and this in turn depends on the mother's health, diet, physical constitution and whether she smoked. A low birth-weight baby, particularly one who is 'small for dates', is likely to be less responsive and energetic than babies of full-term and normal weight. She may take longer to develop the communicative skills we are concerned with in this book – particularly if she is in an incubator where the parents have restricted access to her – but most pre-term babies catch up well during the first year.

Immediately after birth, the baby has to cope with things and events for which she has no previous experiences or frame of reference to draw on. While she was inside her mother's body, she was taken care of, provided oxygen, food, kept warm and protected. Now, at birth, all this changes dramatically; she must learn to take care of herself. The baby must suck and swallow food, digest it and excrete its wastes. Additionally, she must cope with stimulation such as light, sound, voices and being handled from the world around her. In order to be able to cope with these stimulations, the baby already has a number of skills which she can activate.

Posture and movement

Immediately after birth a baby is capable of a number of movements. Some of these may be very complex and others are less so. You can test this for yourself: for example, if you touch her at the corner of her mouth, she will turn to the same side in an attempt to suck your finger.

This behaviour is much more than *reacting* to the stimulus of your touch; it already involves co-ordinated movement and perhaps, more importantly, represents some form of anticipation or *expectation* – namely, wanting to suck your finger. She will make many different movements in response to contact from you. If you gently scratch her down one side of the spine, she will curve her back. She will grasp objects or fingers placed in the palm of her hand. Her hand-gripping reflex is powerful enough to actually support her own weight, but this strength will disappear temporarily, to reappear later in a more purposeful way.

You may have noted that in whatever position you place her, she will curl herself inwards with her body taking up its position in relation to her head. The baby arranges herself 'round her head' in this way because the head is so large and heavy in comparison to the rest of her body. Human babies have large brains to enable them to accomplish the prodigious feats of learning that they achieve in the early months and years – but their bodies, unlike

Meeting other members of the family.

those of other young mammals, are comparatively immature.

The neck muscles at this stage are not very strong, but within a week or so after birth she can begin to control these muscles, enabling her to lift her head away from you (or towards you) but only for a few seconds and only if you hold her against your shoulder. Overall, the baby's voluntary movements are restricted until her muscles and nervous system develop fully. This motor development normally starts from the top, with the baby controlling her head, and then moves downwards and outwards until the baby is capable of balancing and walking on her feet and making delicate movements with her hands and fingers, as she will in her second year.

One group of muscles that the new baby *can* control well are the eye muscles. Although babies cannot at first move their heads or bodies very efficiently to follow moving objects or people, they can – and do – move their eyes in a purposeful way, as if to work out where things are going and where they will reappear. If you lie or prop your baby where she can see things coming and going – by a window, for example, or within sight of moving toys such as mobiles, or other children playing – watch her eyes. You may well find that she is concentrating quite purposefully on some of the activity going on in front of her. This is why it is a good idea to let your new baby be upright sometimes, either over your shoulder or on your back, or propped comfortably in a baby-seat, so that her eyes are not staring at the ceiling, but are able to focus on interesting things and actions.

Newborn babies have other motor reflexes, such as 'walking' when they are held upright on a flat surface, which disappear after a few weeks, only to re-appear much later when conscious control of these movements is possible.

Sucking and feeding

Sucking behaviour, as already mentioned, occurs before birth. The behaviour is quite complex and involves a sequence of movements indicating a precise and innately-organised co-ordination. Sucking involves swallowing and breathing and this will occur spontaneously when the baby is awake and in contact with something suckable, although babies can also suck and feed in their sleep. Your baby may do so on and off all night if you have her sleeping in the same bed with you, without disturbing you. On the other hand, you may find it is very difficult to get her to suck, even when she is in contact with the nipple.

This problem requires specialised help from an understanding midwife or other helper and great patience and perseverance from you, if you are a breastfeeding mother, as it can be a source of long-running feeding problems. This is distressing for both of

...*recognising the breast*...

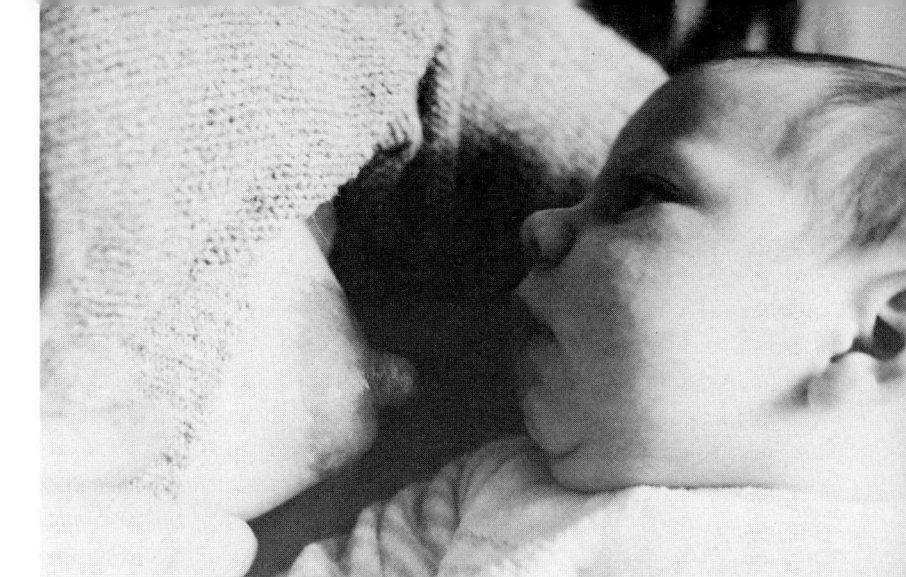

...*his eyes open wider*...

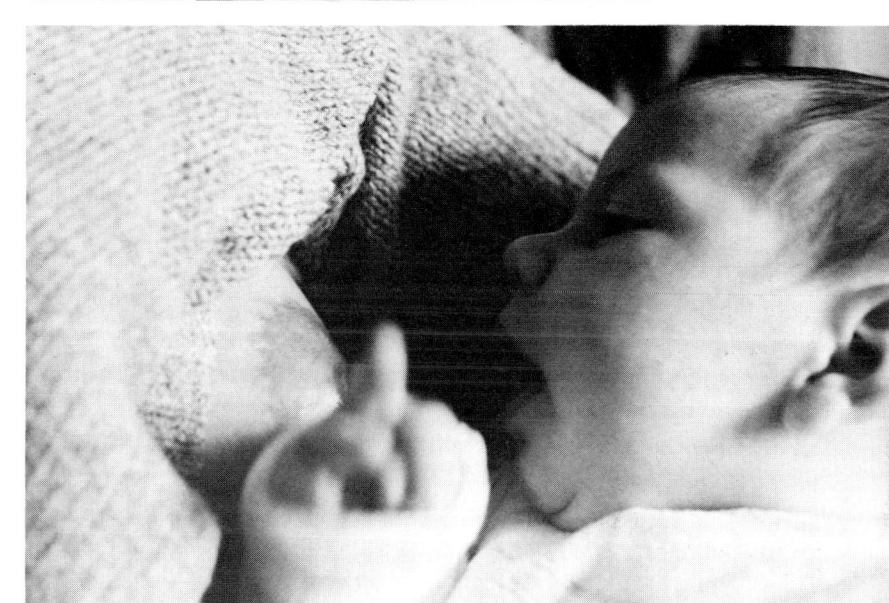

...*and hurls himself at the breast*...

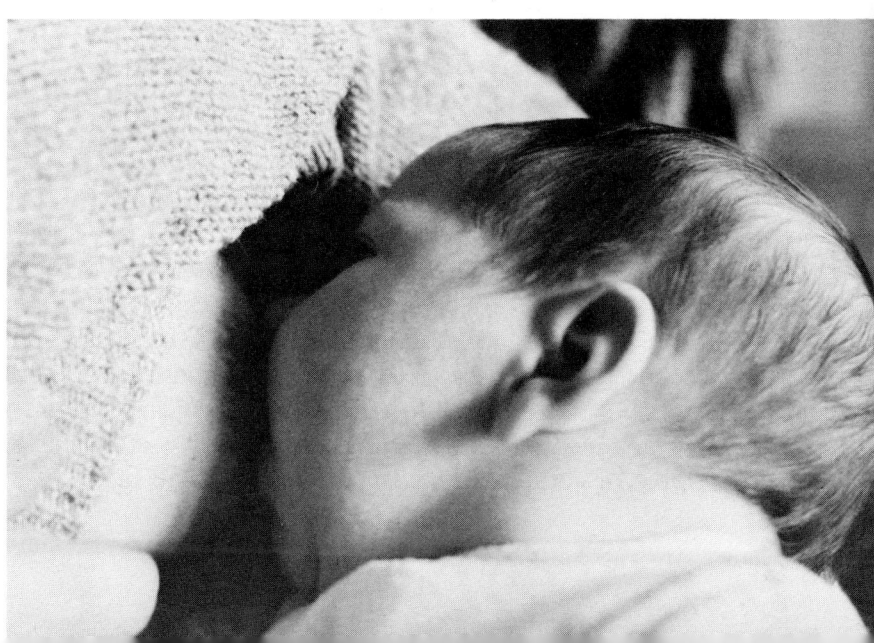

you, not least because it can interfere with the establishment of your relationship and the enjoyment of the many pleasant interactions which should take place during happy feeding sessions.

Studies on the behaviour of mothers and babies during feeding have noted that sucking is organised (primarily by the baby herself) into a 'burst-pause' pattern, with the number of sucks per 'burst' varying from about five to twenty and the pauses between bursts varying from four to fifteen seconds.[16] It looks as if sucking behaviour is already adapted to social interaction and the 'stop-start' nature of her sucking provides you with the opportunity to talk and play with her in the pauses. This sensitivity of each partner to the other, with polite 'taking of turns', is the basic component of all relationships, and it begins to happen when your baby is only a few hours old.

Feed-times are thus very important as a way of getting to know each other and as the opportunity for your baby to hear your voice, be exposed to language and to begin putting what she *hears* together with what she is doing and what she is seeing. You will also learn from her about what sort of sounds or touches she likes; when she wants to 'converse' and when she just wants to get on with the business of feeding with eyes firmly closed. Because feeding is also learning and relating, it is not a good idea to leave your baby propped with a bottle, or to hand her round to lots of different people to feed (a loving dad or sibling is different). If you are breastfeeding, of course, this dilemma will not arise, although breastfeeding mothers can get distracted into reading a book or talking to others because breastfeeding is so easy and automatic, once it is established. Although there is no need to gaze devotedly at your infant throughout each and every feed, it is important to remember that feed-times are especially geared to conversation and attention and should thus be enjoyed together as much as possible.

Sucking has also been used as a way of demonstrating other skills in babies. The co-ordination they can show between different kinds of perception and response was illustrated in an ingenious study using a kind of electronic dummy.[17] By sucking a dummy linked to a device that controlled the clarity of a picture, the babies could either make the picture clear or blurred. The babies consistently sucked more to produce clear pictures rather than blurred ones. The striking element was the way the *looking* behaviour of the babies was combined with the consequences of their sucking: first they looked; then they made the connection between what they could see (clear or blurred) with what they were doing (sucking). They then modified their sucking to produce what they wanted to see – a nice, clear picture. This is a clear example of very early intellectual activity. The other very important aspect of sucking, from the point of view of language development, is that it exercises and strengthens the muscles of the mouth and jaw – and this is essential for clear speech.

Sound

Babies can hear very well soon after birth. Indeed, there is evidence that they can hear noises from the outside world while they are still in the womb.[18] When they are born, they are confronted with the task of sorting out all the many and various sounds they hear all round them: voices, music, heartbeats, loud, frightening noises such as doors banging, domestic noises, traffic and so on. There is ample evidence that they soon begin this sorting-out process.

One psychologist, working in a delivery room, noted that babies just a few seconds old could turn their eyes to a sound source, either to their right or left.[19] This implies something more complex than the ability to locate sound. Turning the eyes towards the sound source suggests that the baby was expecting to *see* something at the source of that sound. This suggests that the newborn baby already has the ability to co-ordinate information coming in through different senses and to know that sounds come from something or someone with a visible presence.

Other studies show how newborn babies can discriminate between different sounds. Researchers have shown that babies can be quickly 'taught' to turn their heads to the right whenever they hear a high-pitched tone, in order to obtain a drink.[20] When they heard a buzzer, they had to turn their heads to the left to get the drink. It required only a few attempts for the newborn babies to reach a state of perfect discrimination, knowing exactly which way to turn their heads, depending on the sounds they heard. This sensitivity to sound-differences is obviously crucial in the development of speech.

Other evidence (see Chapter 6) has shown that babies aged from twelve hours to two days can move in synchrony with speech. At this early stage, the babies moved synchronously with the speech whether it was English or Chinese! Later on, as described in Chapter 5, they begin to sort out the particular sounds belonging to their own language and to ignore others. Babies expect voices to come from mouths and are puzzled and distressed by experimental set-ups where this does not seem to be happening. They also associate sound with touch (as they associate sight and touch in the case of interesting visual presentations) and will reach out towards a noise in the dark.[21]

The development of perception

A newborn baby receives information through all her sensory systems and will respond differently to new sensations. Touch, sound and sight (at this stage still limited to a focusing distance of about nine inches) all tell her what kind of a world she has been born into and give her ways of exploring it and eventually manipulating it herself. Touch gives her warmth and comfort and alerts her to cold and pain; sound tells her that people are nearby and it can also give comfort, particularly when it is rhythmical; light (which she had little experience of in the womb) illuminates everything around her. You may notice that your baby likes brightness and will turn her head towards a light – but she dislikes very bright lights. Even with her eyes closed and when she is asleep, she will screw up her eyes and tense her muscles if a bright light is suddenly shone into her face. This reflex allows her to orientate herself towards the source of the light and allows her to control the amount of light entering her eye from that source.

New babies soon come to prefer face-like images to other similar kinds of round shapes – as a number of studies have shown.[22] Mothers usually become convinced that their babies *know* them after only a short time. It seems likely that the baby learns to know her own mother by a combination of voice, appearance and smell (another important sense – new babies show preferences for pads smelling of their own mothers rather than pads belonging to other mothers).[23]

Your face is probably the first clear unblurred vision your baby experiences and will continue to do so whenever you feed her, hold her or talk to her. Faces are associated with food, comfort and stimulation, and as shown in later chapters, eye-to-eye contact which begins at birth plays a very important part in the development of language.

New babies can also learn to enjoy looking at other things and discriminating between different kinds of shapes and patterns. There is evidence that they like looking at complex patterns rather than simple ones, even when these patterns are only stripes compared to patches of plain grey.[24] These experimental findings indicate that your young baby is capable of making fine discriminations between different kinds of visual presentations and of showing her preferences. So do not be surprised if your baby becomes bored and fretful if she only has the same blank wall or ceiling to look at all the time. If you give her a change of view, or put some interesting mobiles within her range of vision, she will probably become interested and absorbed. Again, remember that boredom can set in if she only has the *same* toys to look at – but there is no need to bombard your baby with elaborately constructed bits of equipment. Faces and the scenes of everyday

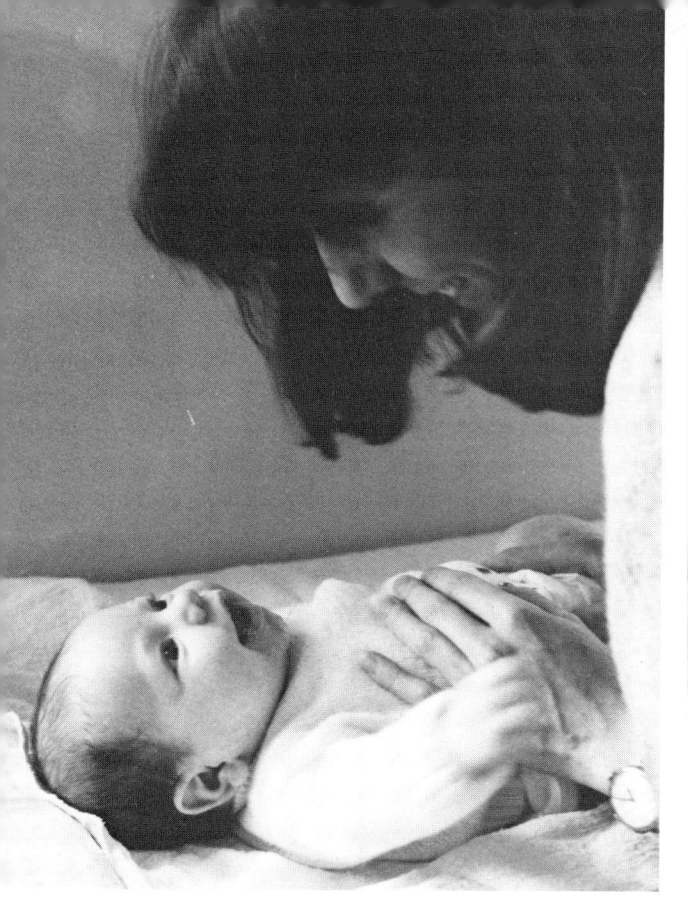

'Hello, what are you doing?'

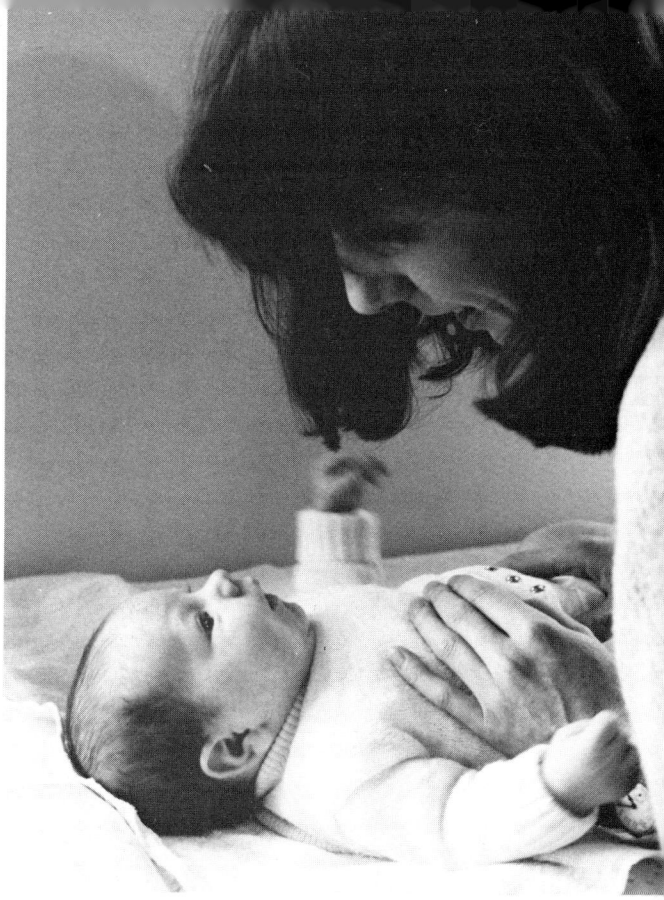

'Oh, wanting to pull my hair?'

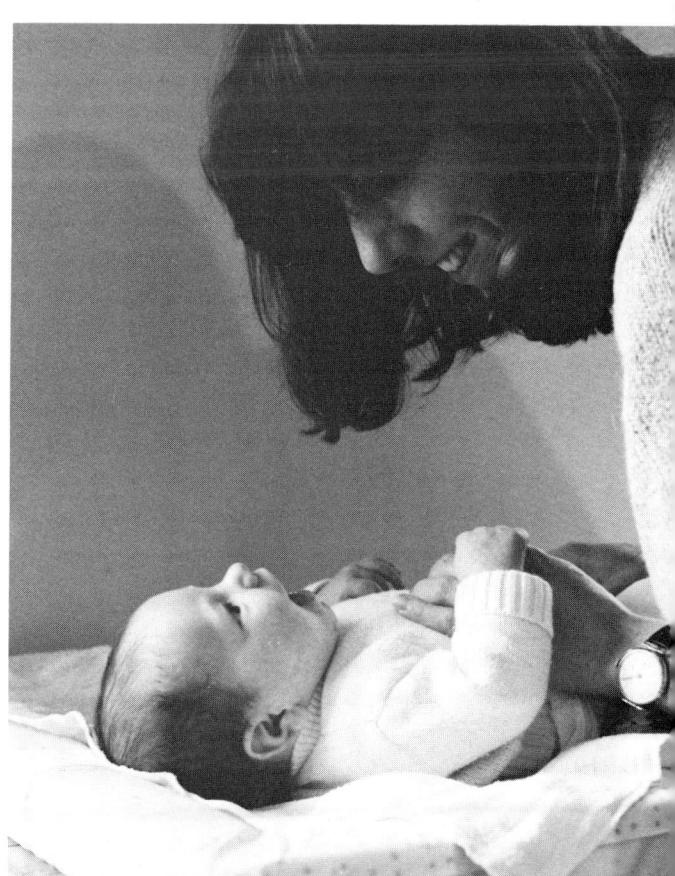

'What a lovely smile'

life provide plenty of variety, so keep her with the rest of the family and take her out as much as possible.

If you want to *show* your baby something, it is best if you show her the toys or pictures at about a nine-inch distance as this is the range of visual focus for a new baby. (It is approximately the same distance as your face is from hers when you breastfeed her.) You may find, after a few weeks, that she tries to reach and grasp – babies expect to be able to *feel* what they can see. Such early exchanges between you and your baby are obvious occasions for language learning. Reaching for an object is a way of *asking* about it. You may reply verbally: 'Yes, here's your bell. Listen to it ringing. Clever girl' (as the baby grasps it), and so on.

Absorbing the world

A great deal of learning goes on during the newborn stage, and during the next two years your baby will build on each new piece of information, each new skill that she acquires to extend her physical, intellectual and emotional range further and further. These two years are a period of very dramatic and exciting development in your baby; they have been labelled the 'sensori-motor' period by the Swiss educator, Jean Piaget, because the child learns primarily through her senses and through movement, although of course there is no abrupt end to this stage, and she will go on being 'sensori-motor' after this.

The stage begins with the newborn's capacity for simple reflexes and very limited purposeful actions and ends when language and other symbolic ways of representing the world appear. This means that the child not only acts – she can represent these actions mentally. She can think about her favourite toy when it is not there and she can refer to it in conversation. She not only enjoys playing a game with her daddy; she can remember it and ask for the same game the next day. Bricks are not only nice solid blocks of wood that can be sucked and banged; they can be turned into cars, houses, boats, slices of bread.

One of the most useful ways of measuring your baby's progress in this direction is looking at how she acquires the notion of 'object permanence'. This means that she understands that a toy exists when it is out of sight; that the same toy can be at the same place at different times or in different places at different times and still be the same toy. It also involves learning that any one object can only be in one place at one time. The stages of reaching this understanding are shown in the chart on page 137. These are only guidelines as babies differ very much in the rates at which they develop. Most children, though, however fast or slow they are, will have fairly similar abilities at twenty-four months.

You can use these guidelines to play with your baby. Try hiding

Learning through games: the toy is hidden – but the child knows where to look.

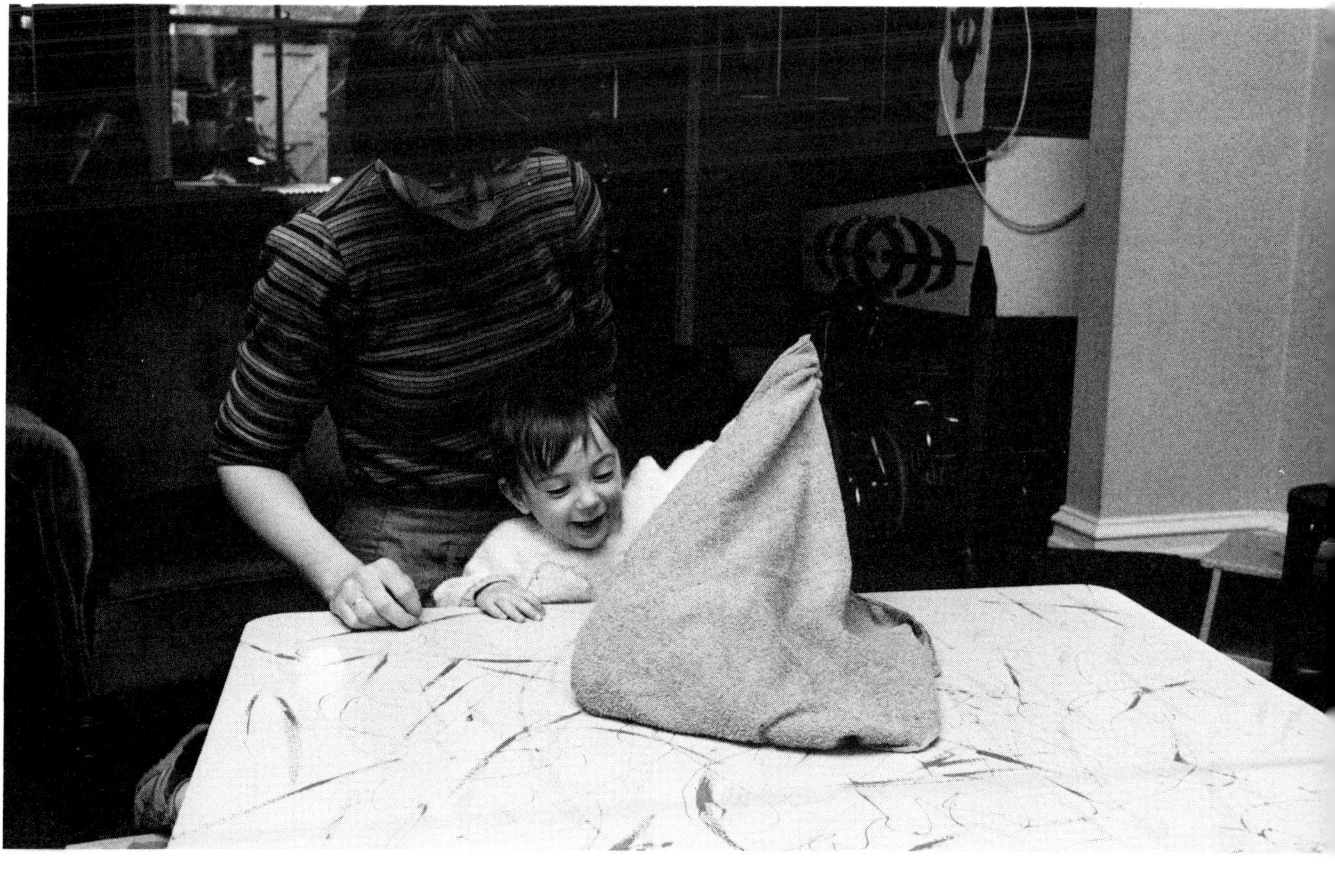

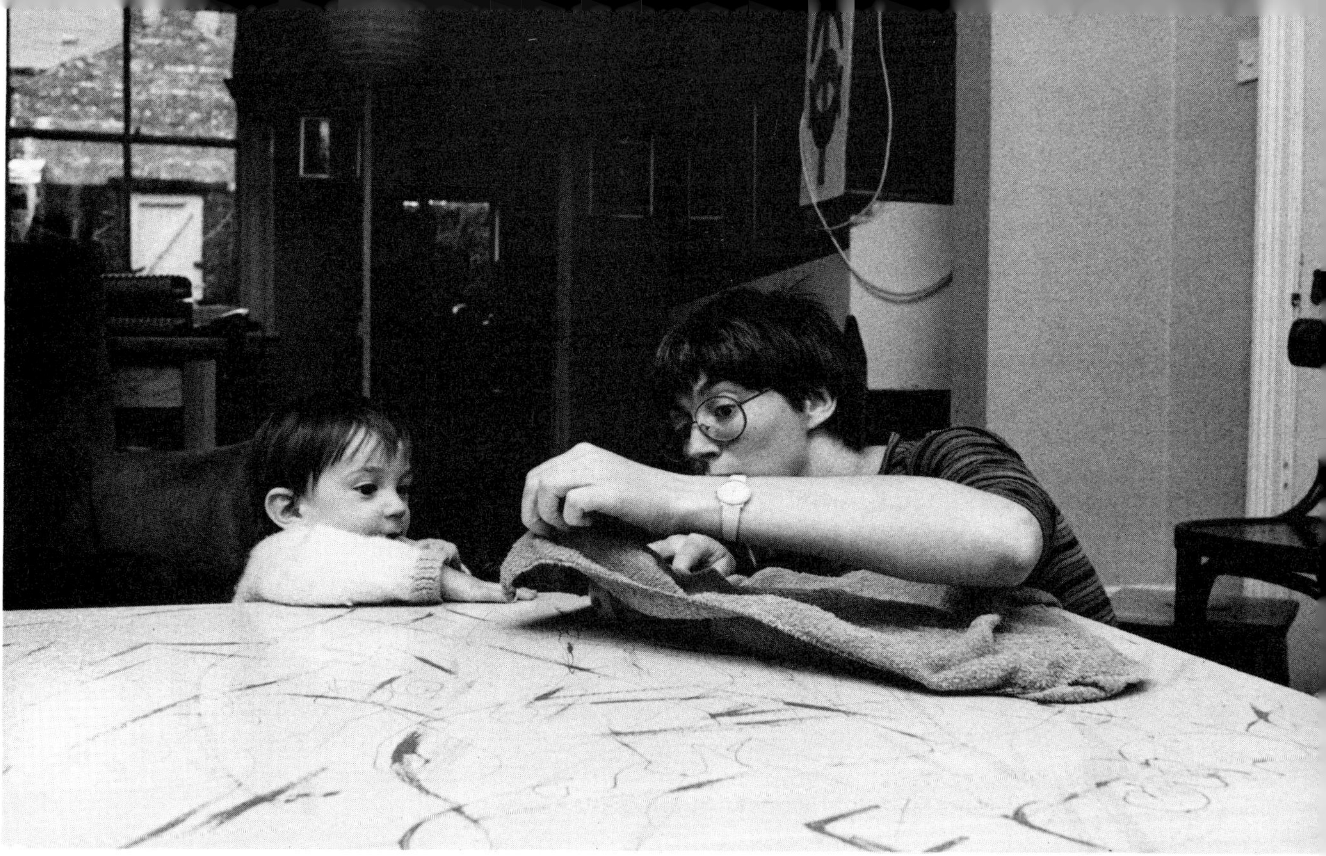

35

something under her chair and see if she leans over to look for it in the correct place. Try hiding a brick under one of several cups and see if she picks up the right cup in order to find the brick. Try hiding it under the same cup a number of times, and then put it under a different one. Which one will she go for? The one where she has already found the brick successfully a number of times? Or the new one? Babies love games that involve disappearing and reappearing, such as peep-bo. Older babies, who can grasp things effectively, love putting things into containers and taking them out again. They have a natural fascination for 'intellectual' exercises like these: 'What happens if I put this beaker inside that one?' 'If the ball rolled under the sofa, will it still be there if I look for it later?' 'If mummy disappears behind a blanket, when will she come out again?' By playing such games with her, you are not only having fun but exercising her problem-solving skills too!

You can read more about the many fascinating developments that take place during the first two years in some of the other books mentioned in the Booklist on page 132 – and of course you can learn most of all by watching your own and other people's babies. As far as language is concerned, it should be clear that the 'symbolic function' described here is a very important part of learning to use language effectively. Once your baby realises that things and people still exist, even when they are not there; that actions can be both mentally remembered *and* anticipated ('Where *did* she put the toy? My guess is it *will* be under there.'), she will begin to see the usefulness of a set of abstract symbols to express these discoveries and ideas to the people she cares about. These symbols are called words.

3
Crying

'When I was a student I heard all about "the competent newborn" – but when I had her, there was no competence about it. All she did was cry.'

Baby at birth: Newborn babies cry – it is their main means of communication.

These are the rueful words of Nicola, a psychologist, who had recently given birth to her first baby. Her comment makes a very important point about newborn babies and the way they in-

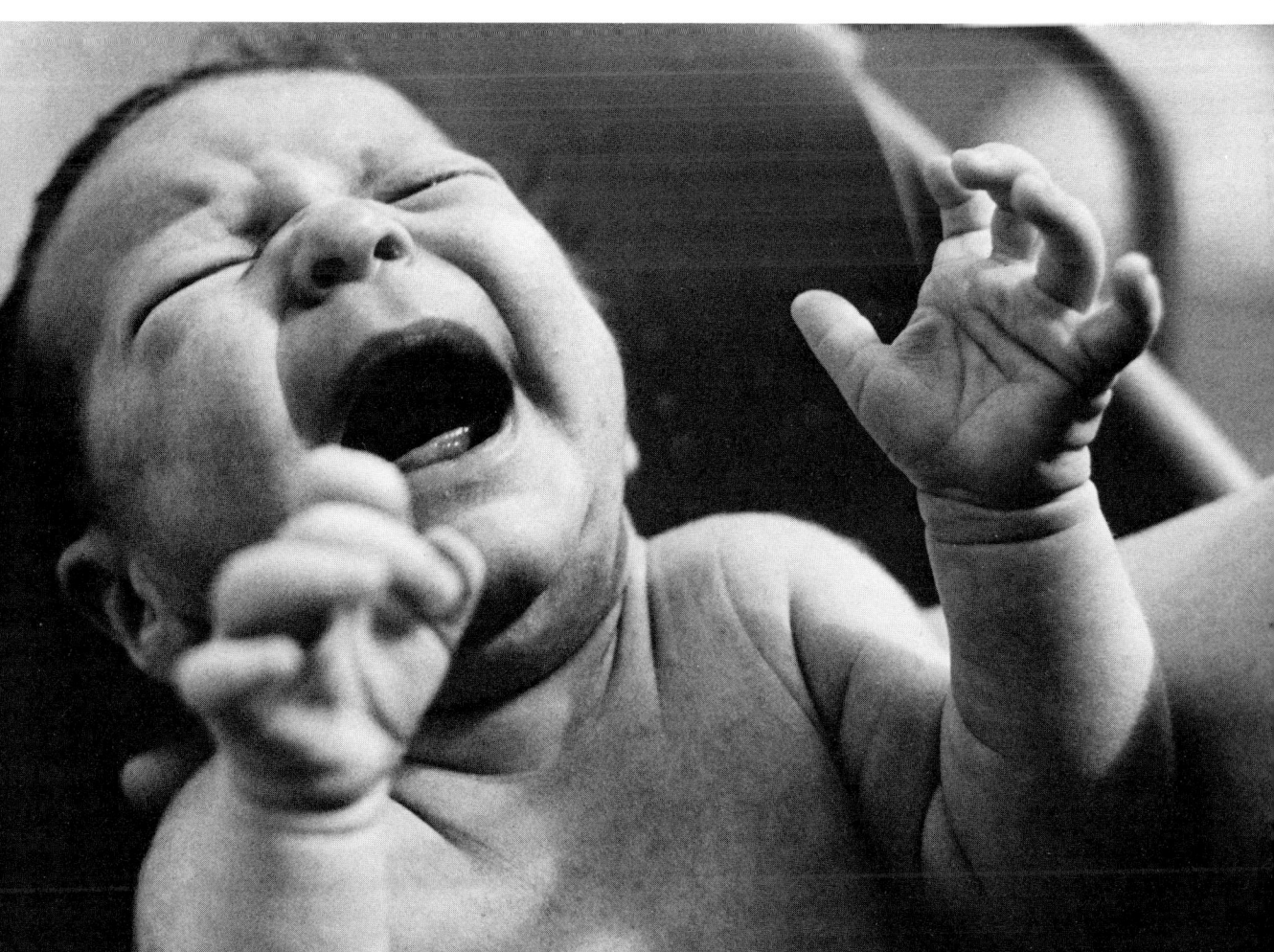

fluence the adults in their lives. In fact, crying is quite a 'competent' thing to do if you are a baby; it is a guaranteed way of bringing someone to your side who will meet your needs. But from the mother's point of view, crying can be very disturbing, especially when, as with very young babies, it is hard to know exactly *why* the baby is crying. A first-time mother, particularly, will not stop to think coolly and calmly about why the baby might be crying; she will not speculate analytically about the efficiency of the baby's signalling system. She may simply feel overwhelmed by a feeling of inadequacy because she cannot understand the baby and she does not know what to do.

Understanding the baby's cries

Different kinds of cry can be distinguished, even in very young babies. In one study,[25] tape-recordings of the birth cry, a hunger cry, and a pain cry were played to experienced nurses and mothers. These nurses and mothers were able to distinguish accurately between each type of cry. Sophisticated recording equipment can produce traces of the different kinds of cry and these printouts do look distinctly different from one another.

However, you will not have sophisticated recording equipment in your home. You will have to rely on intuition and experience in recognising different kinds of cry – and this can take time to acquire, especially if you have a baby who cries a lot, whatever your efforts to soothe her. However, it can be done, because your baby, and your own increasing knowledge, will give you other clues about the causes of crying and what to do about them.

The first cry

When a baby is born, it is vital that she starts breathing through her mouth and nose and hence through her lungs in order to get oxygen into her body. Even a short delay in the first breath can cause permanent brain damage. When a baby cries at birth, air is taken into her lungs and expelled again; she is breathing. Everybody is relieved and can relax.

The first cry is thus a signal for rejoicing among the parents and medical staff at the birth. It can be a prolonged yell, or it may be a few whimpers, or one sharp squawk. The midwife will usually aid the process of introducing air into the lungs by sucking out any mucus that the baby may have in her throat. The first real cry may follow this process.

Some people have argued that the first cry is a cry of pain and protest at being born into a harsh world. The French obstetrician, Frederick Leboyer, has described this first cry: 'The tragic expression, those tight-shut eyes, those puzzled eyebrows . . . That howling mouth, that burrowing, desperate head. Those outstretched hands beseeching; then withdrawn, raised to the head in the classic gesture of despair . . . So can we say that a newborn baby doesn't speak? . . . Could this little creature already be a person? Suffering? Howling with grief?'[26]

Not everyone would agree with this interpretation of the first cry. Nor, indeed, do all babies behave in such a 'desperate' way. Partly thanks to the influence of Leboyer himself, many births these days are conducted in a calm, peaceful atmosphere. The baby will be delivered straight onto the mother's body and into her arms. The baby will probably cry, but is unlikely to scream with 'despair', unless, of course, she is uncomfortable for some other reason.

However, Leboyer's somewhat rhetorical question, 'Could this little creature already be a person?' can be answered with the word 'Yes' – as the kinds of studies described in Chapter Two have indicated. Something that mothers have long felt intuitively – that their babies *were* individual human beings, that they *could* feel, that they *could* learn, that they *could* recognise their own special caretaker – now has the support of carefully-gathered evidence. As a result, you will probably be encouraged to treat your baby as a person and when she cries, you will recognise this as a sign of distress that needs comfort, just as you would with any other person.

Your baby should not cry for long after birth. Ideally, you should be able to nurse her at the breast (if you are breastfeeding); this not only soothes the baby, it is a vitally important first step in establishing successful breastfeeding. There is evidence[27] that the sooner a baby is put to the breast after birth, the more successful breastfeeding is likely to be. And if feeding goes well from the start, this, in itself, will reduce the chances of frequent crying later. Other observations of babies at birth, for example by Aidan McFarlane in Oxford[28] and by the American paediatricians, John Kennell and Marshall Klaus,[29] have shown that many babies are actually very calm and alert immediately after birth. If you are feeling well yourself, the hour or two after birth can be a good and happy time for getting to know your baby and building a good foundation for your relationship, which, again, may lessen the likelihood of miserable behaviour in the future (on both your parts).

If you are *not* well yourself – perhaps because you have had a difficult forceps or even Caesarean delivery, or a long, exhausting labour – you may not get off to such a good start. The baby is also likely to be affected by a difficult delivery. Indeed, emergency procedures are used precisely because the baby is showing signs of distress. There is evidence that babies who have had difficult births and whose mothers have received a lot of medication are more likely to cry a lot in the first year.[31] Of course there is not much you can do about this once it has happened. But if you did have a difficult delivery, and you have a baby who is fretful, understanding *why* she is fretful and realising that it is not your fault can help you to feel less guilty and anxious about her crying. This can take some of the tension out of the situation and may improve matters generally. After all, if you feel guilty and anxious, your tension may communicate itself to your baby and contribute yet more to her fretfulness. If you relax, she may cheer up. And even if she does not, at least one of you is feeling better.

Reasons for crying

Many people think that babies, particularly newborn ones, cry only for straightforward, physical reasons: they are hungry, or cold, or wet or in pain. If you feed them, keep them dry and warm and put them in a cosy crib, they should be happy. Unfortunately, quite often they are not happy and either start crying or continue to cry. A fascinating study of eighteen babies during their first month, which was carried out in the United States by Peter Wolff and his colleagues, observed and recorded the occasions when the babies cried and experimentally tried out some of the reasons that the experimenters thought might *make* them cry – though, not of course, to the point of extreme distress.[32] The experimenters also studied some of the techniques that caused babies to stop crying and these gave important clues as to why the babies were crying in the first place.

From the first week onwards, these experimenters found that there were *psychological* reasons, as well as physical ones, for babies crying. In other words, tiny babies, like other people, cry when they are upset about something, not just because they want feeding or covering. They also found, as many parents of more than one child discover, that there are individual differences between babies: what upsets one baby may not bother another.

Some of the babies were followed up to the end of their sixth month. As you might expect, the reasons for crying changed as the babies got older, and hence, so did the techniques for getting them to stop. Increasingly, the baby's 'frame of mind' when the cause for crying occurred influenced how much she cried, or not. If a baby was in a good mood, she would show interest in a toy or a person or a sound. If she was already crying, she could not be cheered up by the same toy or person or sound. In fact it would annoy her. So, if your baby is really hungry or uncomfortable and is yelling hard, diversionary tactics will not work. Babies can't be 'fobbed off' when they are determined to be picked up or fed.

Hunger crying

During the first few weeks, hunger crying has a very distinctive, rhythmical sound: cry, breathe, cry. The American researchers compared recordings of this cry with other cries – a 'mad' or 'cross' cry, in which the babies seemed to be mildly annoyed about something, and which did not particularly distress their mothers, and a 'pain cry' which followed a heel-prick (the Guthrie test) and *did* distress both mothers and nurses. The different cries produced very different recording patterns.

The problem with the hunger cry is that it also occurs at times other than when you think the baby is 'due' for a feed. It can occur perhaps only an hour after the last feed. What do you do then? Other researchers have found that the response to a cry can very much depend on the mother's reading of the situation. If you are a demand-feeder, you will pick up the baby, even after only an hour, and feed her again. If you feel she should have been satisfied by her last feed, you may try other techniques for getting her off to sleep or soothing her. If she is your second child and you're occupied with your first one, or you know from experience that babies sometimes spontaneously stop crying and doze off by themselves, you may leave her until you are ready to respond to her.

Some people think that if you always respond to a baby's cry, whether by feeding or comforting, you encourage her to cry more and more; she'll be 'spoilt'. In fact, the evidence suggests that this is not how it works; babies whose parents respond to them sensitively and promptly will probably in the end cry less.[33] However, this is not an infallible rule; many very sensitive and capable parents have babies who cry whatever they do. In this case, it can be hard to maintain your confidence in yourself as a good parent. It may help to remember the point that babies differ very much as individuals; the fact that your baby cries a lot is *not* a reflection on you. It may be that she is just a miserable baby. (Babies that cry excessively are discussed in more detail later in this chapter.)

The most appropriate response to the hunger cry, once you have learned to recognise it, has to be feeding. The American researchers found that hungry babies could not be satisfied by sucking alone, although it might keep them quiet for a few minutes. In the early weeks, it is usually easier to respond to regular, rhythmical crying by feeding. If you are breastfeeding, this is important as a way of stimulating a good milk supply. However you feed, remember that being picked up and nursed, even if only a little milk is taken, is the easiest way of providing comfort too. As the baby gets older, you will find other ways of comforting her that are more suited to her developing abilities; a baby who wants to be amused by company or play should not always be 'fobbed off' with a feed. Try a cuddle and a conversation for a few moments to see if this produces a calming effect.

Pain and discomfort

The pain cry, as Peter Wolff and his American research team found, was the most disturbing to adults. The recordings showed that it always had a sudden onset – no whimpers, moans or gurgles leading up to it, and the babies held their breath for a long period between each cry. These cries were observed when the babies were given a routine blood test which involved a heel-prick. Obviously, at such times, you will expect your baby to shriek and you will do all you can to comfort her afterwards. Once the pain has gone and you have comforted her, the crying will cease.

If you hear this sudden, urgent kind of crying when your baby is at home with you, check her for sources of pain. The proverbial nappy pin is supposed to be rare in practice, but it can happen! She may have got herself into an uncomfortable position in cot or pram; her clothes may be tight for her; there may be an uncomfortable lump under her. When they are older, of course, the occasions when babies hurt themselves multiply. A mobile crawler and toddler can bump herself, fall over, tread on something sharp, or cut and burn herself on ordinary household objects. To prevent these kinds of pain and distress, you will have to make your home safe.

If you cannot find any obvious reason for your baby or young child screaming in pain, you must get your doctor to check her; she may be ill. Earache is very common at night, in a child who is otherwise well during the day. Stomach pain may indicate an infection which should be treated. If your child is too young to tell you where the pain is, an expert professional examination is even more essential.

A very common cause of painful crying in babies under three months is *colic*. The baby produces the characteristic pain cry, which is very disturbing to you, and draws up her legs over her stomach. The symptoms of colic appear to indicate severe stomach pain, but the mysterious aspect of colicky crying is that it usually only occurs at a certain time of day. It can be late afternoon or evening. It occurs in both breastfed and bottlefed babies; some babies never have it at all whatever they are fed on. It is thus difficult to decide what is causing the stomach pain – if stomach pain it is. Some breastfeeding mothers have found that cutting cows' milk and other dairy products out of their diets has stopped their babies crying with 'colic'. This seems to indicate an allergic problem. But this does not apply to all babies. You can try this solution, with your doctor's approval, and see if it works for you.

Sucking a dummy and warmth applied to the stomach may also help. Wrapped in a shawl, lay your baby on her back on your lap, holding her legs in the air and gently but firmly massage her lower abdomen. If you have a colicky screamer do seek advice; you can also contact the Cry-sis! organisation (see Useful Addresses on page 131). Try to get a break from the baby sometimes, too. Colicky babies are nearly always very healthy babies, so there is no cause for worry. Letting someone else listen to her for a while can give you fresh energy for the next day. Colic usually passes by three months.

Wet and cold

People sometimes think that babies are crying because they want their wet or dirty nappies changed. The American researchers tested this idea and found that it had little foundation in truth. Some of their crying babies were changed from wet to dry nappies; the others were picked up and 'changed', but the wet nappy was put back on. Babies in both groups stopped crying. It seemed that it was the attention of being picked up and changed that the babies wanted, not the relief of dryness.

However, none of the babies liked being cold very much. Some disliked it more than others. When the temperature in their cribs was lowered from 88–90°F. to around 78°F., the babies were more likely to wake up and cry. Perhaps for the same reason, many babies – particularly between the second and fourth weeks – protested at being undressed. Being undressed, of course, also involves being pulled about quite a lot and, if you are still rather inexperienced, you may find getting vests and baby-stretch suits on and off yelling, slippery babies quite unnerving.

To lessen the trauma, make sure the background temperature of the room is *very* warm – at least 70–75°F. Undress the baby on a soft, warm surface, such as a lambskin rug or soft shawl, if you feel insecure with her on your lap. Cover her over with a warm towel or blanket if she has to be left naked while you do something else. Do not leave her on a cold, hard plastic or rubber surface. Both the research and the experience of many mothers show that babies are happier when they are close to something soft and warm; this can, of course, be you. Cuddling your naked baby close to your own warm skin (perhaps after *your* bath, or during a breastfeed) can bring great contentment and enjoyment to you both. Close skin contact like this applies equally well to fathers as well as to mothers. Contact comfort seems to be something that babies need almost more than anything else – even more than food sometimes. So do not be afraid of picking your baby up and cuddling her, or of enjoying this experience.

Frustration and fear

One of the earliest psychological reasons for crying seems to be frustration. The American researchers found that being deprived of a dummy and the enjoyable sucking experience it gave, caused even newborn babies to cry with irritation. They also cried at the interruption of a feed. The 'frustration' cry was a variant of the pain cry, but not so acute.

The researchers also identified an 'attention-seeking' cry from about the third week onwards. This consisted of long moans, developing into full cries and back into weaker moans. This kind of crying was relieved by voices and other sounds and by being picked up. In recent years, a great deal of research has been done into the intellectual abilities of very young babies and it has demonstrated that, almost from birth, babies enjoy having things to do. They like making things happen, such as producing noises from bells and rattles hanging over them. They can attempt to reach out and grasp things in their field of vision; their quest for knowledge and stimulation has already begun. If babies have no sources of knowledge and stimulation – nothing to do, or look at, or listen to, or expect – then they will be bored and fretful. The frustration or attention-seeking cry will call you to them.

If your baby seems to be crying in this non-urgent way and does not want to be fed or go to sleep, you may find that carrying her around, or propping her in a baby-chair where she can see other people and reach interesting objects, will stop her crying.

You may be told that you should resist this need for attention, as if attention, unlike food, were an unreasonable demand for a baby to make. But if you accept that your baby is a person, a need for attention is no more unreasonable than it is in any other person. Nobody likes to be ignored. Babies are limited in what they can do for themselves. Giving your baby attention and amusement will be more enjoyable for both of you than 'making her wait'.

During their first six to eight months, babies will cry from hunger, cold, annoyance, frustration, boredom, loneliness and pain. But it is very unlikely that they will cry from fear. The concept of being threatened by something unfamiliar and hence disturbing develops later and is actually a stage in your baby's intellectual progress. At around eight months, she will have worked out who and what belongs in her familiar world and who does not. Anything or anyone that does not belong is grounds for suspicion and if familiar people go away and leave her with someone unfamiliar, or if she is put in a very unfamiliar situation, she will become anxious and is likely to cry.

Stranger anxiety usually develops at around eight months, but signs of it can be detected earlier. At around two to three months, your baby may protest at being left by any person – not necessarily just you. If she has a special familiar cuddly toy she may object if it is taken away. Young babies may also show puzzlement and distress if your appearance changes for any reason, but it has to be a fairly drastic and distorting change. The Wolff researchers found that six-month-olds were not frightened, even when their caretakers wore masks. They *were* upset, though, when their mothers, who usually wore spectacles, took the glasses off. Oddly, when mothers who *did not* usually wear glasses put some on, their babies were not upset. So it is not quite clear what kinds of distortions are most upsetting to babies.

What is clear is that, as they get older, they become more attached to what is familiar and safe and more likely to cry and be made anxious by the strange and new. Again, there will be individual variations. Some babies will happily go to strangers, even after the eight-month 'watershed'. Others may show great clinginess towards their mothers at a much younger age. Hannah, aged two months, screamed with protest when her mother left her on her grandmother's lap to go to the telephone. She calmed down as soon as her mother returned and picked her up. This 'clingy' trait persisted until she was nearly two years old.

Anger and protest

We have already mentioned that both mothers and researchers were able to identify a 'mad' or 'cross' cry in babies only a few weeks old. This cry did not seem to indicate any particular need; the babies just seemed irritated with themselves. Young babies often cry like this when they are tired but cannot get off to sleep; you can help them settle down by firm holding, wrapping or by rocking. (More techniques that work in getting babies to stop crying and to sleep are given later in this chapter.)

Frustration, for example, when dummies are removed, and protest at being left alone can also be expressions of anger. But really angry crying and yelling begins to develop most noticeably when your baby becomes a toddler, before she can express herself in words very clearly. From around fifteen months to about two and a half years is the age of the notorious toddler tantrum. The tantrum can be an expression of the child's will and her desire to challenge yours. She will often choose the perfect place for it – somewhere like a shop, or a tea-party at your in-laws', where she can rely on you not to lose your own control in case other people disapprove.

Tantrums are an expression of anger and frustration and they usually disappear once the child can make her wishes known verbally. They are thus an important, if inconvenient form of baby language. If you can see them as an expression of frustration and

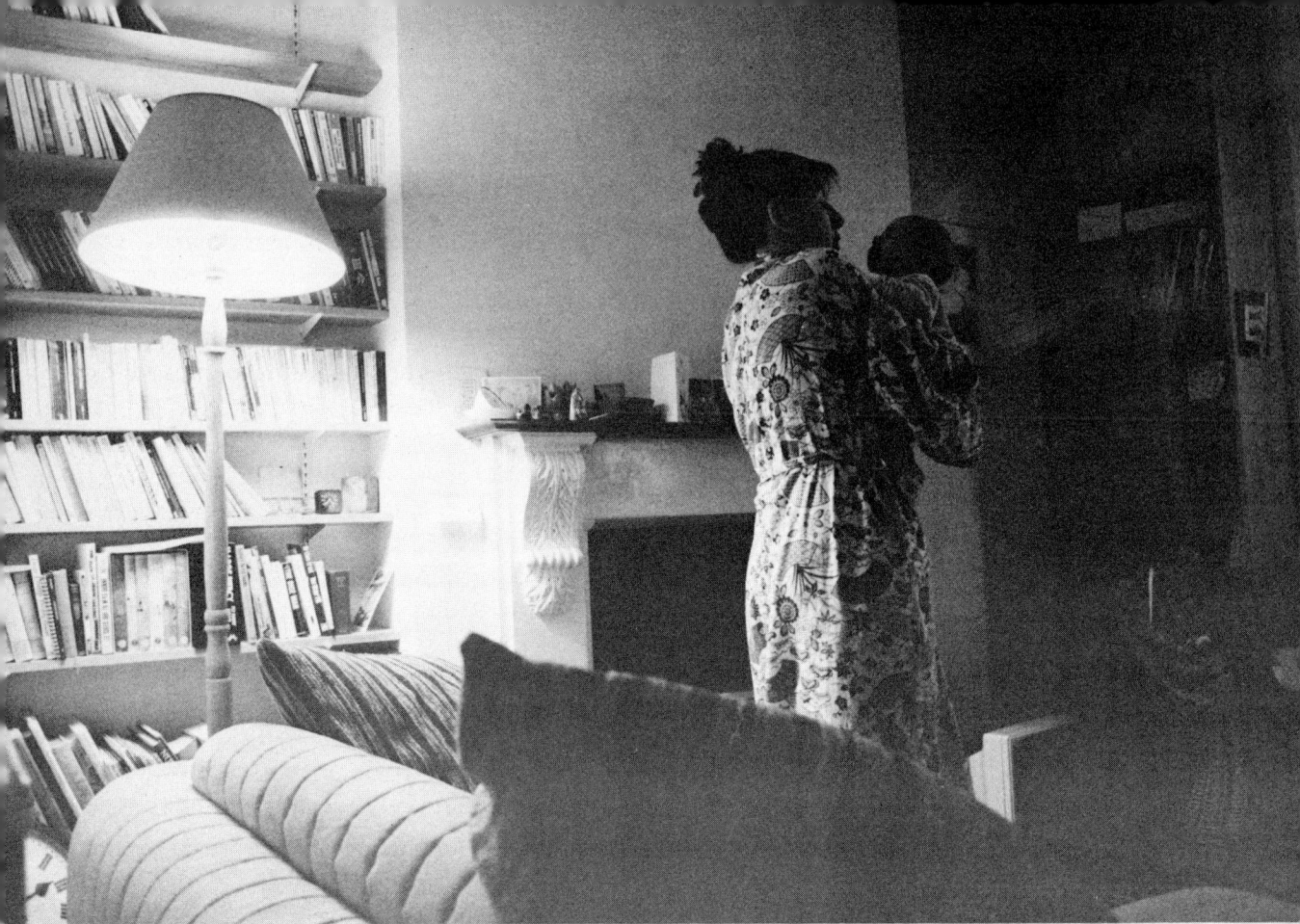

of the inability to communicate, this will help you to be more sympathetic and less threatened by them. Your child is not really being wicked and rebellious to you; she just does not know another way to get what she wants.

However, tantrums do need to be brought under control, for the child's sake as well as everybody else's. Firm holding and, if possible, removal to a quiet place can help. Do not try and match the child's volume or intensity; wait until she calms down and then try to find out what she wants. When you are in public, distraction or bribery *do* help. You might not want to give your child a sweet or a treat if she were behaving aggressively at home, but in public this can be a possible solution.

Preventing outbursts of angry frustration by being aware of your child's needs and weaknesses is the best way to head off tantrums. If you *know* that she is not going to eat egg or drink from a cup without throwing the whole lot on the floor, it makes sense not to give her egg or a cup and to warn people that you are visiting not to do so. It is not worth making an issue over such matters at this stage. Later, when her understanding and verbal skills are greater, you can *explain* that some foods are good for you and that big girls drink out of cups. But such rational

Crying can be very disturbing to a new mother – especially at night.

explanations are beyond the comprehension of most under-twos.

Constant crying

Babies vary a great deal in the amount of crying that they do. One study found that one baby cried for an average of 64 minutes in 24 hours during the period from two to thirteen weeks of age; another cried for an average of only seven minutes in 24 hours. (Of course, these times are averages and individual babies will not cry for the same amount of time every day.) There can be discoverable reasons for these differences between babies. For instance, the kind of birth they had and the way their mothers responded to them has an effect. But some babies just seem to cry a lot, regardless of their experiences or the sensitivity of their parents.

If you have a baby who cries nearly all the time, regardless of how often you feed or comfort her, the first thing to do is check with your doctor that she is well. Check, too, that she is not reacting to anything that she is eating or that you are eating (if you are breastfeeding). When you have ruled out possible physical causes for her crying, you need to take steps to cope with the crying and to learn to live with it so that it does not totally disrupt your family life and relationships.

A positive first step is to contact another parent who has been through the same problem. The Cry-sis! organisation (see Useful Addresses on page 131) can put you in touch with such a sympathetic supporter. These mothers stress the importance of getting a break from the baby sometimes. Try to go out together as husband and wife, leaving the baby with a trusted relative or friend. Do as much as you can to relieve other pressures; if you have other children, see if you can get friends and babysitters to look after them occasionally. It can be worth economising on other things to get some paid help with housework. You may qualify for a home help; ask your health visitor or social services department about this. Do not feel guilty about asking for help: you will be of little use to your children if your own nerves are in shreds and you are physically exhausted.

If your baby cries at night, try taking her into bed with you – and do not feel guilty about giving her a dummy. Try to catch up on your own sleep with brief naps during the day. Keep a diary about your baby's crying patterns. You may spot regular times when she is particularly fretful and you can arrange your own day so that there are no other pressures at these times. 'Constant' crying does eventually stop – reassure yourself of this.

Crying and speech

Crying is the first *sound* that a baby makes; we think of it as her way of 'talking', but we do not *see* it as proper speech. But there is a relationship between the sounds of crying and the development of other sounds that the baby makes, which eventually become proper, meaningful speech. The Wolff research, which recorded periods before and after crying as well as the cries themselves, found that as early as the third week, babies were beginning to make non-crying sounds, always just before whimpering and then full-scale crying.

At first, these non-cry sounds – gurgles, squeals, raspberries and then little noises such as 'ga ga' and 'da da' – were just a lead-in to crying. But as the babies got older, the babies seemed to learn these noises and to use them at other times, when they were quite happy. Later on, these noises became babbling which is the forerunner of speech (see Chapter 6).

The other noise that babies produce towards the end of their first month is laughter, and this, too, has similarities to their crying sounds. But, of course, it will mean something different to you – it will strike you as a much more pleasant sound. You may tickle and tease your baby in order to produce laughter; tickling can actually be uncomfortable, but the baby produces laughter instead of crying in response to it. Of course, if the discomfort or teasing goes on too long it may end in crying, just as older children and adults can 'laugh until they cry'. Later, your baby will laugh in response to games or funny faces or to enjoyable and exciting activities such as being tossed in the air. Laughter in response to a game such as peep-bo, which your baby will enjoy from around six months onwards, represents a stage in her intellectual development too; she is learning to *expect* that something will happen. Your face, or a toy, will disappear and then appear again; she knows it has not gone for good. She can *remember* it, and *anticipate* its reappearance. The fact that babies enjoy these 'intellectual' games so much shows that they are 'programmed' to learn and to enjoy learning.

Ways to stop a baby crying

There are many ways of soothing a crying baby, some tried and tested by centuries of tradition. Such ways have also been experimentally tested, and it is reassuring to find that many of the techniques devised by mothers, grandmothers and other care-takers are scientifically reliable! Here are some of them. You may have devised others, or your own variations on the traditions. Feeding is excluded from these. It is the only thing that will satisfy a hungry baby. The comfort of sucking and of being picked up can also apply to feeding, but sometimes it is not a feed that a crying baby wants, or you may not be able to feed her there and then.

What do you do?

SUCKING: Non-hungry babies can be soothed by thumb-sucking or by dummies. Sucking is physically enjoyable, but it also has a quality which is important in soothing babies: namely, *rhythm*.

RHYTHM: Sucking is rhythmical. So is rocking – 60 rocks a minute seems to be the optimum rate. A rocking cradle, being pushed backwards and forwards in a pram, being driven in a car, being carried on another person's moving body, all help to satisfy the baby's apparent need for regularity and predictability in her movements.

SOUND: Continuous 'white' noise has been found to have a soothing effect on babies.[34] You will probably find it a little difficult to produce this in your home, but sometimes, if you hold the baby upright and give a high-pitched croon into her ear, you can stop her crying. Some babies like music; other sounds, such as bells and rattles and, of course, the human voice, can also temporarily stop the baby crying. Some parents have found a recording of a heart-beat – 'womb-noises' – successful in soothing crying. You can achieve the same effect by carrying your baby close to your own heart. This gives *contact*.

CONTACT: Contact with another human being is a vital need for the tiny, helpless human infant who can do nothing and can go nowhere without an older person to help her. But it also meets her psychological needs for comfort and for the opportunity to learn. Sometimes a voice and hand is enough; at other times she will want to be picked up and cuddled. A soft, warm surface to sleep on and soft, warm, firm coverings are soothing too. Firmness seems to be important, which is why researchers have found that one of the most old-fashioned ways of handling young babies is also one of the most effective in stopping them crying: *swaddling*.

SWADDLING: Being firmly wrapped up is soothing for babies because it stops them being irritatingly aware of their own uncontrolled movements. Thrashing and kicking around seems to be disturbing and threatening for young babies. The warmth and firmness of swaddling calms them down. (Of course, there will be other times when your baby will enjoy the freedom to kick and wave her arms and she should have the opportunity to do this every day.)

WARMTH: We have already said that babies slept more soundly when their cribs were kept at a higher temperature. Make sure the room your baby sleeps in has a temperature of around 70°F. In cold weather she should be well wrapped up and covered. Cold is

Different ways to comfort a crying baby:

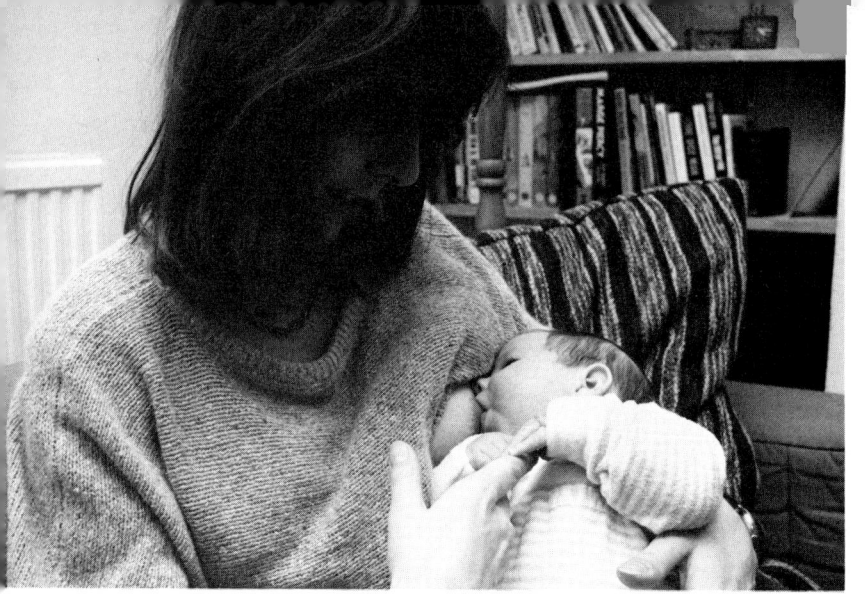

Sucking provides warmth, love and nourishment

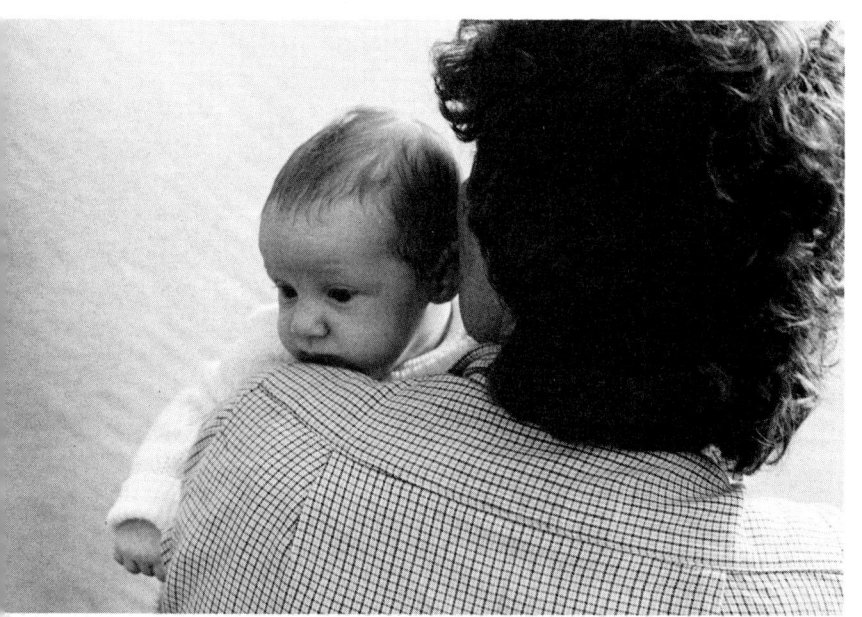

Rhythm is soothing when the baby is rocked

Babies like to be sung to

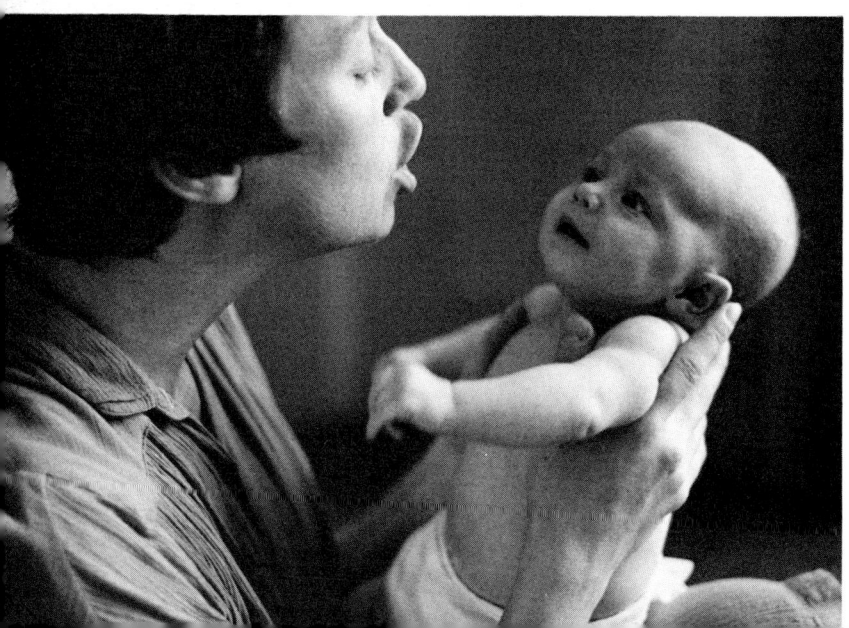

Contact with another person provides reassurance

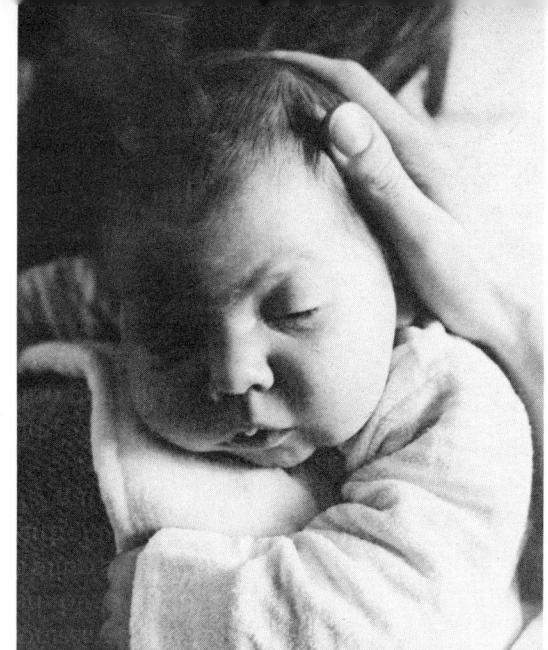

Firm swaddling makes a baby feel secure

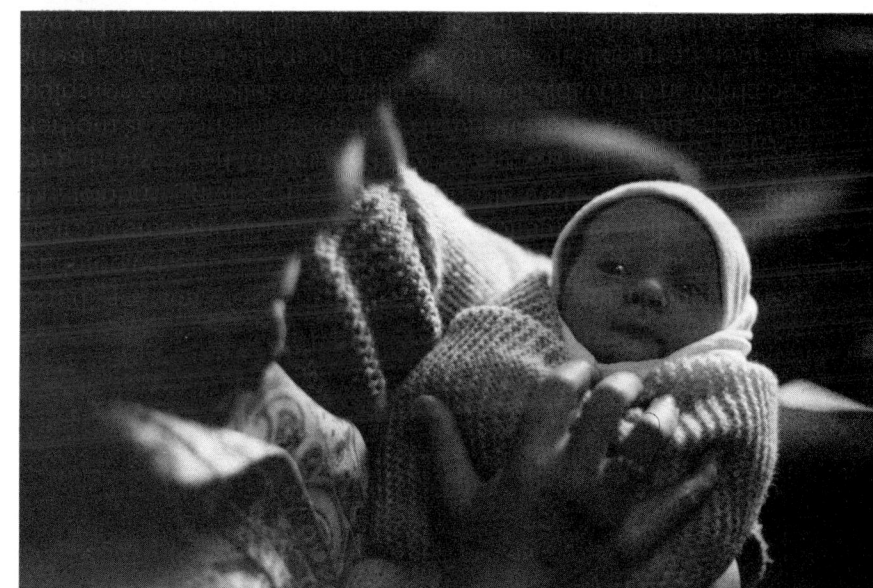

Stimulation and amusement keep babies happy

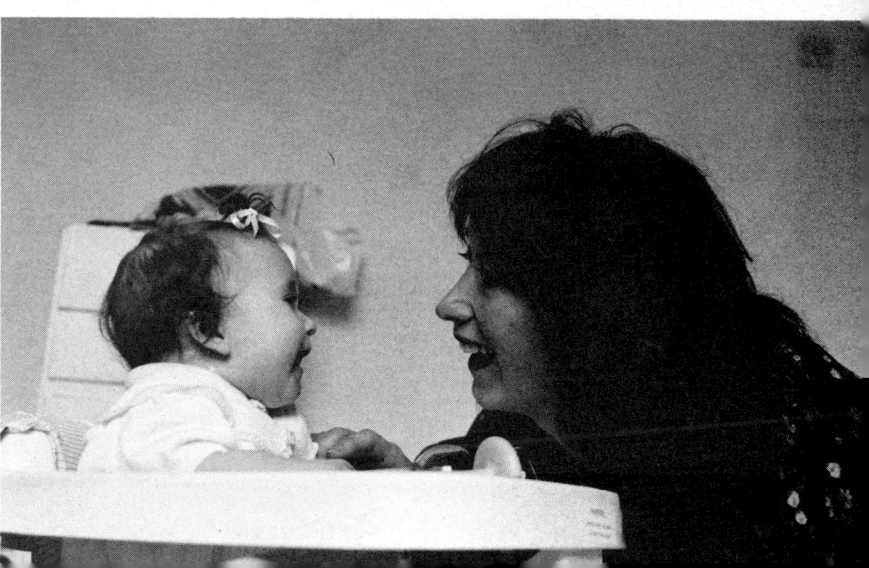

dangerous to young babies who cannot control their own body temperature very well. Again, being carried close to a warm body ensures both warmth and contact. Warmth is essential for relaxing the muscles. You probably know yourself that you become more drowsy and sleepy in a warm atmosphere.

STIMULATION: Your baby will not always want to drop off and sleep. As she grows and develops she will prefer to be amused and to learn. Even newborn babies will stop crying and become more alert if they are held upright over your shoulder where they can see what there is to be seen. Babies like to have things to look at, sounds to hear and objects to hold and explore, when they are able to reach and grasp. Make sure your baby has these opportunities at some time every day. A baby can be over-stimulated sometimes. She may then produce cries of frustration or anger. You can use other techniques – rocking, firm wrapping and soothing sounds – to calm her down and help her to sleep.

As your baby grows into a crawler and then a toddler, her powers of communication will increase also. The time will come when she can tell you what she wants by gesturing and eventually by asking. But crying will go on being an important part of her range of expression. Listening, understanding and responding appropriately to her cries will lay the foundation for the more complex communication between you that comes later.

4

Body Language

> 'Sometimes when I talk to him, he kicks his little arms and legs and his whole face lights up. Other times, he just gazes at me as if he's trying to work out what's going on.'
>
> *Mother, talking about her four-month-old baby.*

When we talk to each other, we use a whole range of signals: as well as the words, to express what we mean. We also monitor other people in order to pick up *their* non-verbal signals: their smiles, head movements, expressions, gestures of the hand that might indicate agitation, or boredom or anxiety. Both partners in the conversation will adjust their behaviour according to their 'reading' of these signals.

This kind of non-verbal communication – or 'body language' – is particularly important for babies because they do not have any words. Yet they have an urgent desire to communicate with others, to gain attention, to make their wishes known and to express their feelings. In the first year of life, particularly, and to a lesser extent as they get older and their spoken language develops, babies use their *bodies* to communicate what they mean and to respond to what other people say and do to them.

Faces

The face is the most sensitive barometer of what is going on either in one person's mind or between two people as they communicate. A newborn baby has a wonderful range of expressions: watch your baby while he is asleep, for instance, and notice how he changes from a look of calm wisdom, to an anxious little frown, to a secretive little smile accompanied by mouth movements as if he were dreaming of feeding, then back to repose. His expressions will also change when he is awake, but at first it is difficult to detect why. His expressions do not seem to have much to do with what you are saying, or doing, or the way you look at him.

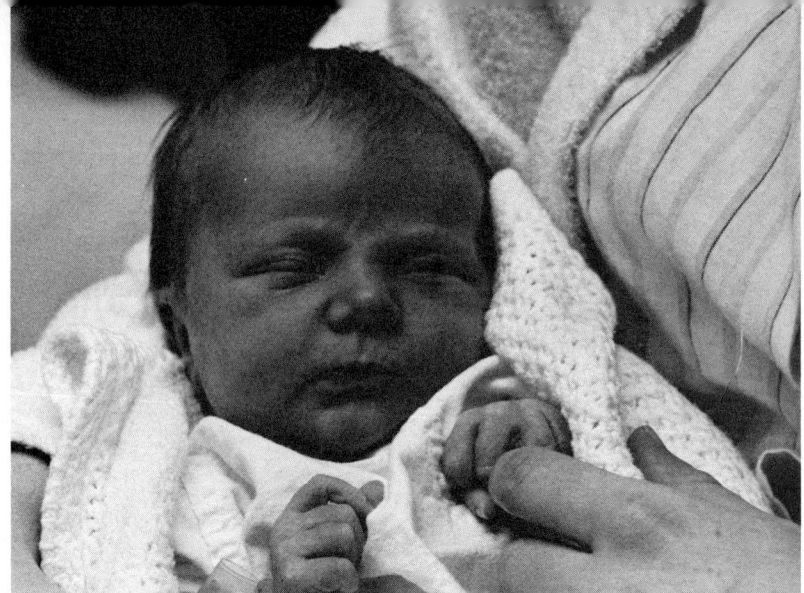

Even very new babies show a wide range of facial expressions

—from boredom

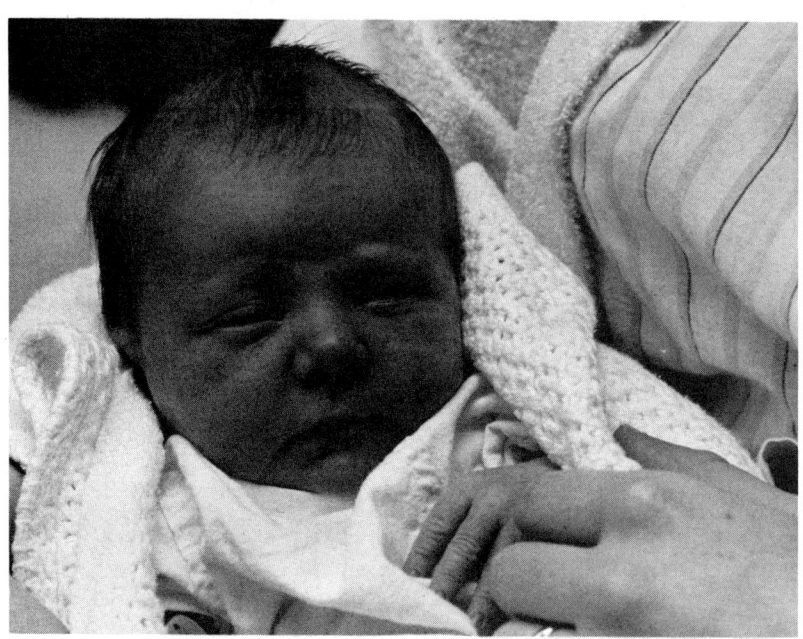

to resignation

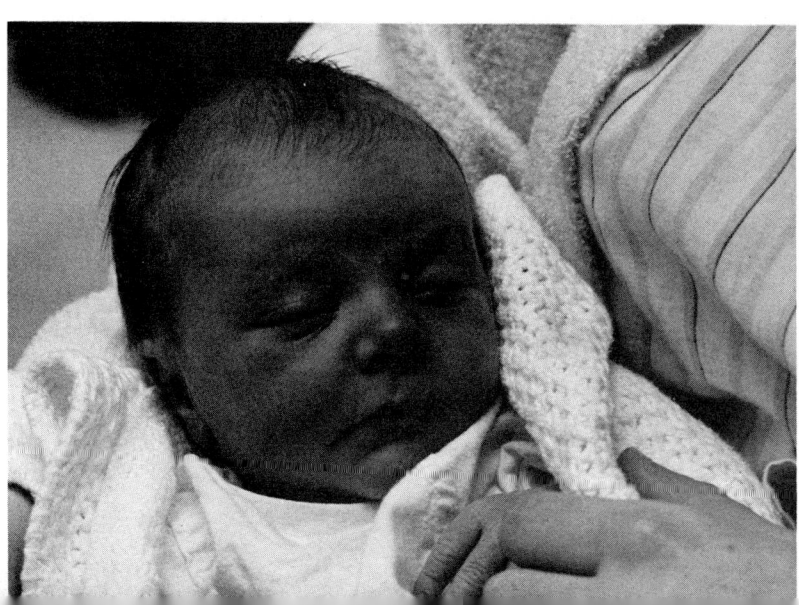

to lofty disdain

quizzical

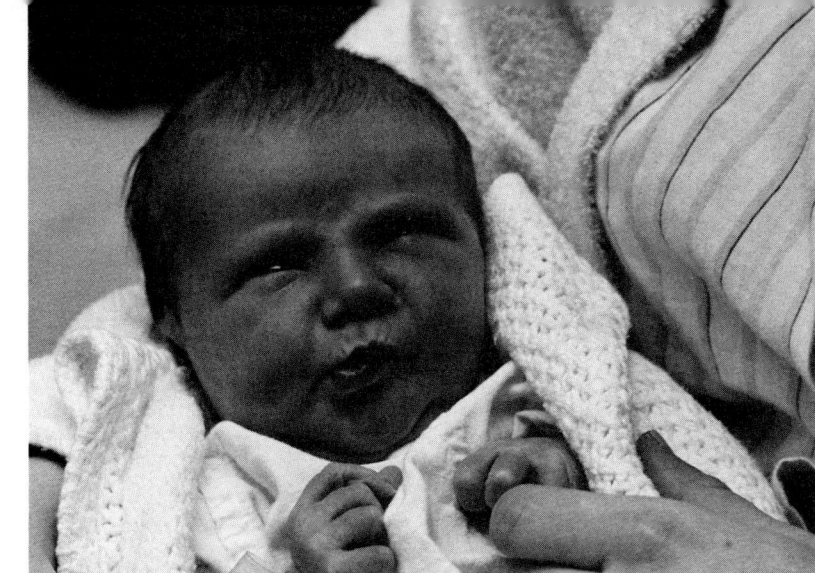

sleepy

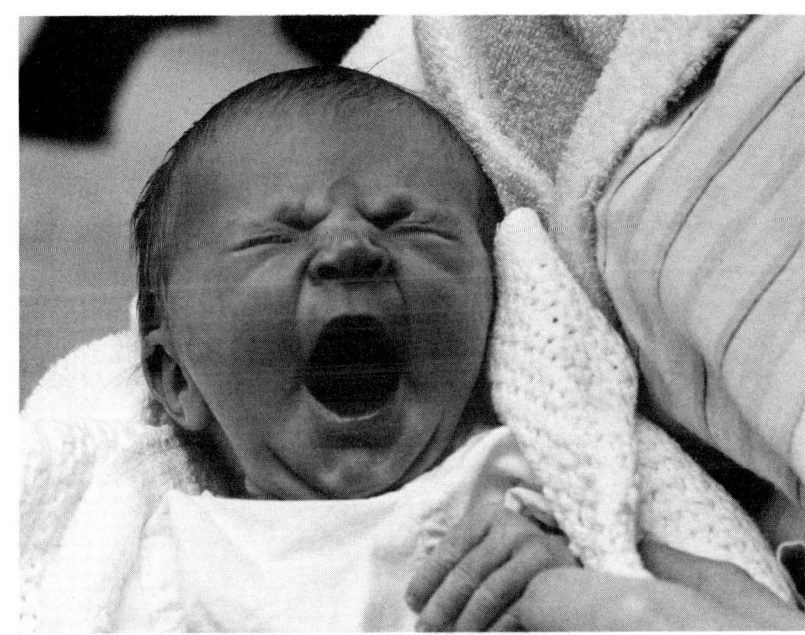

grumpy

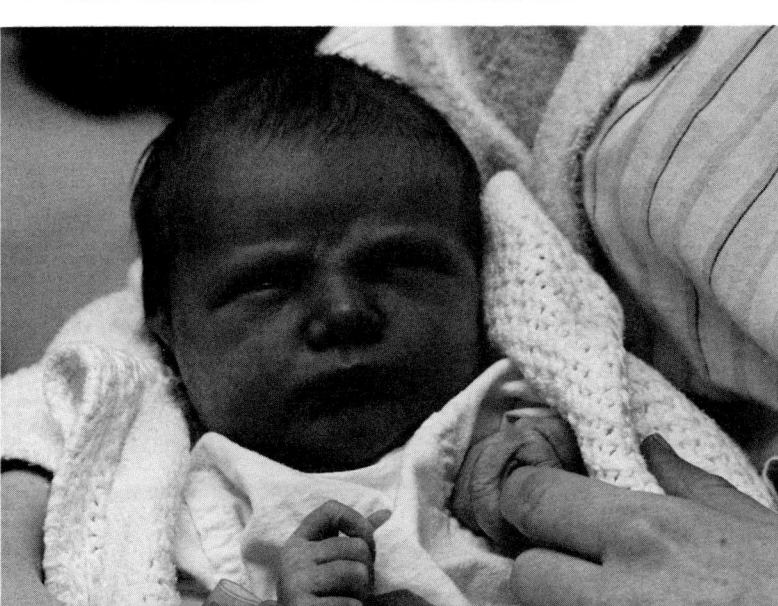

Very quickly, however, within a week or two of birth, some of his expressions will seem to you to be *responses*. He will gaze intently at you when you talk to him; if you turn away, or alter your tone of voice to talk to somebody else, he may look distressed and then cry. If he tastes something unpleasant in his mouth, he may look disgusted. If, on the other hand, he sees the bottle or breast approaching, his eyes will open wider, he will pant excitedly and hurl himself at the nipple with what looks like passion.

Your baby will also monitor your facial expressions. Experiments have suggested that young babies prefer to look at faces (or images of faces, or even just face-like patterns) more than anything else.[35] Your new baby will come to prefer looking at your face, or the faces of other special people, such as father or brothers and sisters, to looking at people's faces in general. There will eventually come a time (around eight months) when strange faces fill him with alarm, but during the early months, the human infant seems to find all faces fascinating. Some research has suggested that the infant is so sensitive to facial expressions in the mother that he can actually imitate them.[36] For a young baby to be able to put his tongue out at his mother when she puts her tongue out at him is actually quite a complex thing to do. At only a few weeks old, he has to know that he owns a face similar to the one that he is looking at and that special movements are required to produce a protruding tongue. How does he know? There are all kinds of scientific arguments about this, and some people suggest that the baby is not really imitating. The mother is probably more likely to be imitating him. However, what matters from your point of view is that you and your baby share similar ways of behaving which can be learned from each other.

Smiles

The first real moment of pure communication between you and your baby is the baby's first smile. Until then you have been guessing about his needs; he cries, you feed him, he seems satisfied, so you assume he was telling you he was hungry. But when he looks at you and you look back and he suddenly flashes a brilliant smile straight at you and you smile back, there is no guesswork involved: this is direct communication and it creates immense pleasure for both of you. You are hooked, and from then on, you will work very hard to produce that moment again.

Peter Wolff, who did the research on crying described in Chapter 3, has also studied babies' smiles.[37] He found that he could get babies to smile during the first week in response to particular sounds, such as whistles and voices; but they only

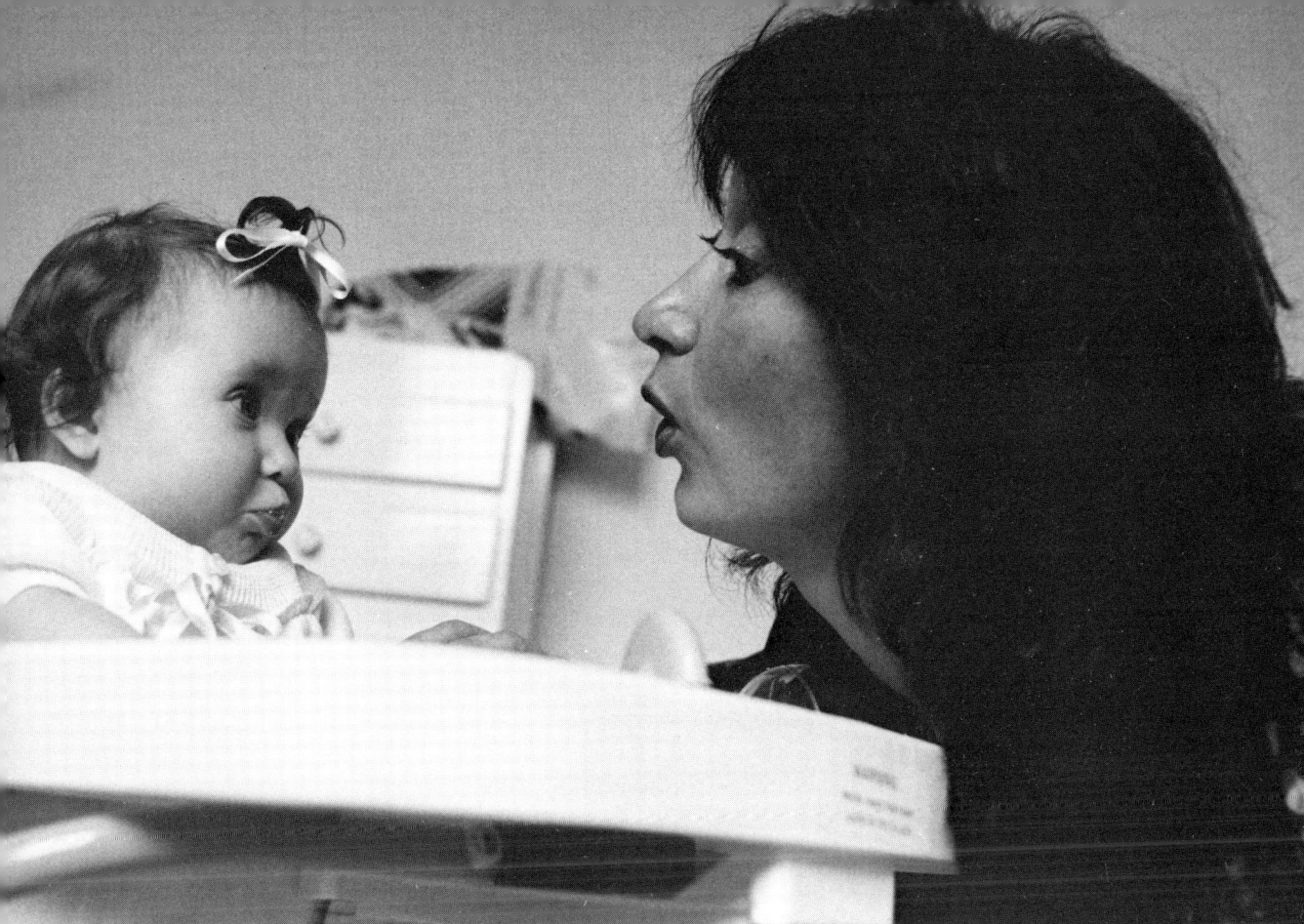

Baby and mother imitate each other: how does she know how to do it?

smiled in their sleep. In the second and third weeks he observed something that you have probably noticed with amusement yourself: babies often smile in a drunken way when they have just finished a feed. Wolff found that he could *make* them smile with his special sounds when they were in this state but not at other times. In the fourth week, he observed the first real smile. This was different from the earlier smiles in that the baby was alert and awake and the smile was a result of direct face-to-face contact with the mother. He suggests that it is eye-contact that plays the biggest part in getting a baby to smile; once a baby can 'lock-on' to your eyes and focus his own onto them, he will produce a smile.

Smiling is a big reward for a parent. You will find that you talk, sing, and play with your baby. You will tickle him, rub his tummy, make silly noises, blow raspberries – all kinds of things to make him smile at you. And, of course, all these things are opportunities for language learning.

Eyes

Eye to eye contact between people encourages all kinds of communicative behaviour. For your baby, his visual sense is very

57

important in telling him about the world he lives in and the people in it; he will understand and learn to manipulate what he *sees*, well before he can understand what he hears and begin to translate what he hears into speech. A newborn baby will turn his head to 'look' at the source of a sound and increasingly your baby's looking behaviour will be guided by sounds of different kinds. He will learn to ignore regular, familiar sounds such as people walking around the house, but will quickly turn and look when he hears the front door open and the new, different footsteps of a visitor.

Babies who cannot *see* are handicapped with regard to language development. In the first place, they cannot notice anything until it is put into their hands. They have no choice about the objects that capture their attention as a seeing baby does. So the first stage of language – labelling *things*: 'teddy'; 'bikky'; 'baby'; 'doggie' and so on – will not come so naturally to them. In the second place, their faces register no expression or response to what the adults around them are doing and saying. So it is less rewarding for the adult to give them all the stimulation that comes quite spontaneously from a mother who knows she will be rewarded with smiles, expressions of delight, querying gazes and so on. Specific handicaps are discussed in Chapter 10, but the point here is that *looking* is the natural precursor to talking. When your six-month-old baby leans over the side of the pram, you will look down too and say, 'have you dropped your blanket?' (or 'don't say you've dropped your blanket again', depending on how many times he has done it). In both cases, you are commenting usefully on your baby's action, and telling him, from your tone of voice, how you feel about it.

You may find it instructive to watch your baby's eyes. What do they follow and why? If you give him a choice of things to look at – mobiles, a view from a window, other children playing in the room, a TV screen – what does he spend most time looking at? These will give you clues about what is capturing his interest and what he finds puzzling or intriguing about the world around him. These will be your topics of conversation with him; his gaze is a way of asking a question. You can use your own gaze in a similar way. If you look intently at something, notice whether he follows your attention, or would he rather look at something else? These kinds of visual 'conversations' can be carried on anywhere; walks down the street, shops, parks, other children's homes as well as your own home all provide new topics of interest for your baby to look at and for you to comment on for him.

Movement

We all use movements and gestures to indicate or underline what we mean: we nod, shake or jerk our heads; we point; we wave; we wag our fingers; we make all kinds of complicated gesticulations with our hands; we lean forward or back; we fold our arms; we cross and uncross our legs and so on. New babies do not have control of their movements in the way that older children and adults do; but they can control their eye movements and they quickly learn to move their heads around in response to interesting noises. You will soon notice your baby lifting or turning his head when he hears your voice, or a new voice, or music, or meaningful sounds which suggest that someone is coming, such as a door opening, or that a meal is on the way, such as the rustle of clothing or the sound of crockery.

New babies appear not to have much control of their bodies and limbs. Their movements seem involuntary. But some fascinating films made by a researcher called William Condon indicated that even a baby a few days old could adjust his movements to synchronise with the sound patterns of an adult voice.[38] It was only possible to observe this synchrony by slowing the film right down and by comparing each minute action with the soundwaves of the voice on an audiotape. The two seemed to fit together, as if the baby were moving in time to a kind of vocal music. This is further evidence of the human baby's ability to respond to especially meaningful sounds; it does look as though he is 'programmed' to be particularly sensitive to voices and to be able to distinguish subtle variations in vocal sounds. This ability is obviously important in the acquisition of speech, since so many words *sound* almost identical ('papa' and 'baba' for instance) but mean something different. It is important that the baby sorts out the difference between 'p' and 'b' and research has shown that babies only a few weeks old can make this distinction, even though it will be a few months before they know what 'papa' and 'baba' mean, and longer still before they can use the words themselves.

During the first three to four months, babies gain quite a lot of control over their body movements. They learn to roll over which helps them to get nearer objects of interest. They also learn to reach effectively. When they see an interesting object they can put out their hands, adjust their grip to the appropriate size of the object and get hold of it. (They will usually try to eat it.) Reaching is a big advance in communication. Watching what your baby reaches for will give you many more insights into what interests him and what you can talk about. It also gives you an effective way of amusing him. Babies get a lot of information and pleasure

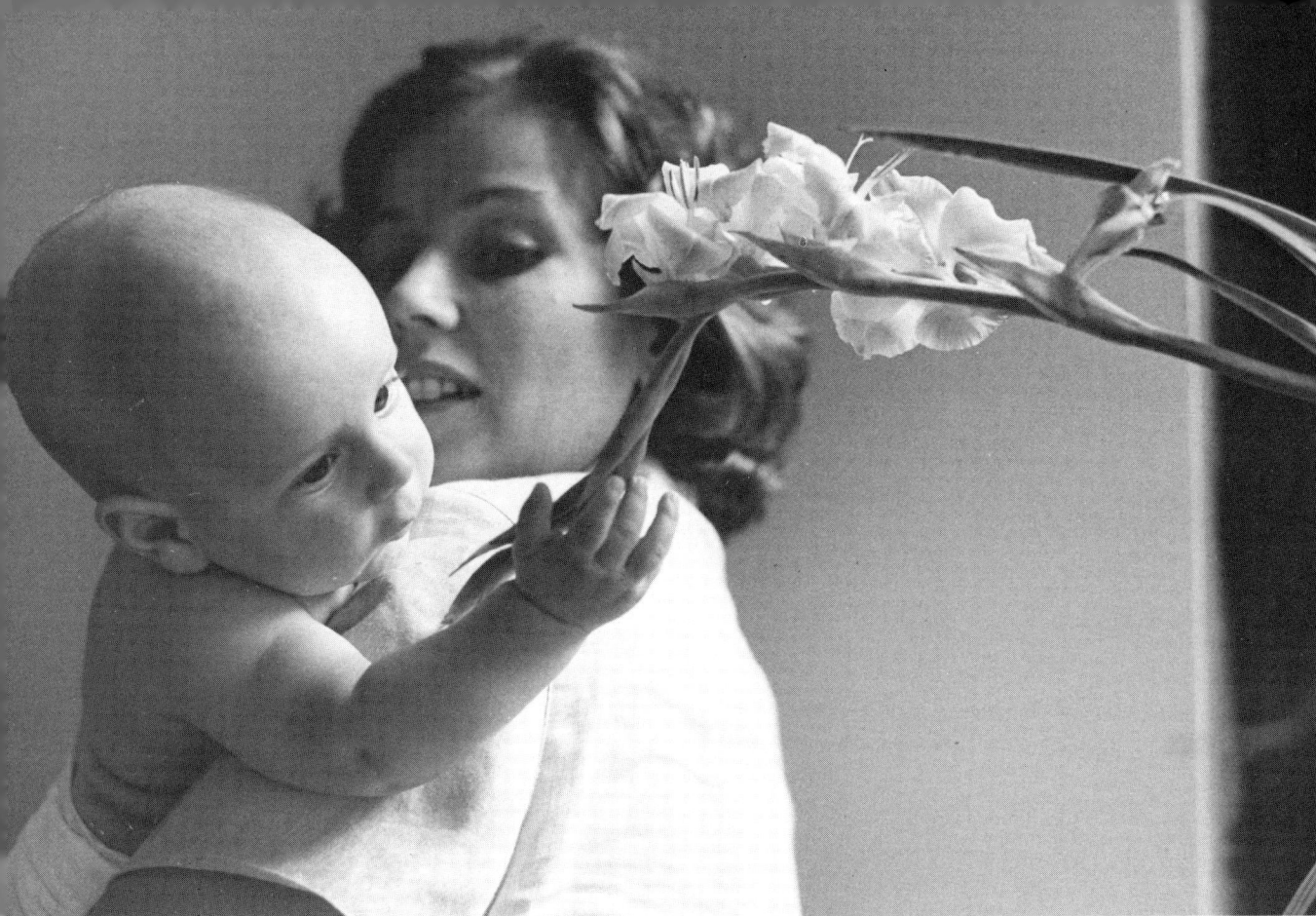

from touching and feeling things. It is a good idea to give your baby access to a variety of different textures and sensations. Watch him on a sandy, pebbly beach for instance; or in an open, grassy space.

All these experiences open up new concepts for him, which will one day be turned into speech: 'The grass is wet'; 'The sand is prickly'; 'Don't put it in your mouth – it's yukky, dirty'; 'Isn't it nice/warm/horrible/cold here?' – and so on. Things not only have *names*; they have characteristics. People are not just objects; they have feelings and sensations. All this begins to be learned before the first word is spoken.

Once your baby can sit up by himself (at around seven to nine months), you will find that pointing becomes a very useful way of gaining your attention and indicating what he wants, or what he is interested in. It will go on being so – even when accompanied by quite effective verbal messages: 'Wassat?', 'Allgone', 'Cat', 'Daddy!' and so on. When he can crawl and, later, toddle, your baby will move *towards* things or people that he is interested in and touch them, or grab them. One researcher who studied his own baby's language development observed that, at eight months, his son had definite 'touch signs' that always meant the

Reaching shows hand and eye working together – and is a way of exploring the fascinating world around her.

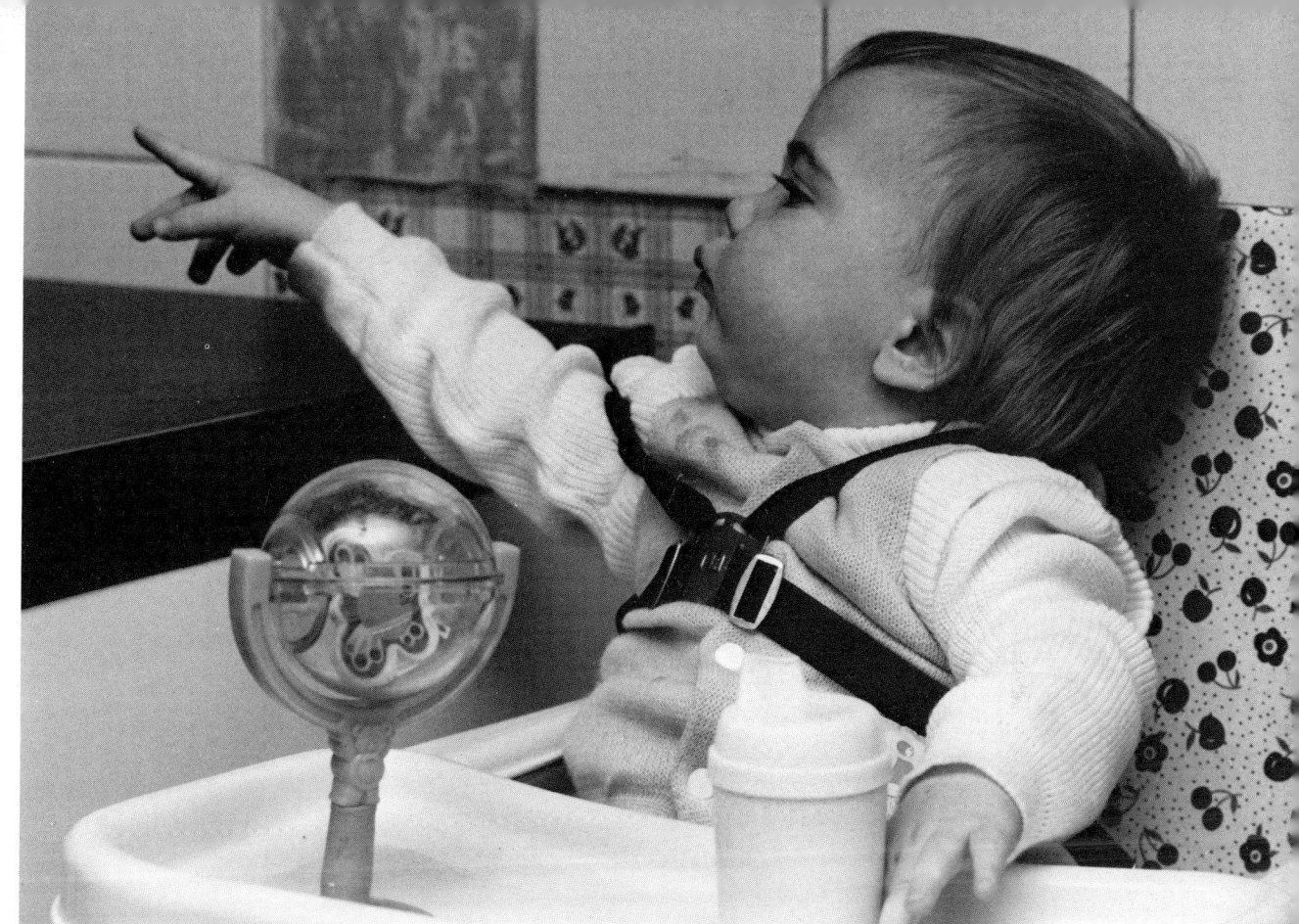

Pointing: 'Look what I can see and I know you can see it too'.

same thing: quickly grasping something and then letting it go meant 'I want that'. Touching something lightly and briefly meant 'I don't want that'. Touching something firmly for a longer period meant 'Do something with that'. You may notice similar signals in your own baby. Of course you can only work out what they mean by trying out a few responses and seeing which one works. If you hand the toy to the baby and he hurls it on the floor, you know he did not mean 'I want that'. It can take time and patient observation to read a baby's signals, but it pays off.

As your baby acquires words and later sentences, the need to watch him and his movements so closely in order to understand him becomes less. But his physical behaviour is still a very important part of learning to communicate. Play, particularly, is a very rich source of language learning. Language is more than just the names of objects, characteristics and feelings. To master it effectively your baby has to acquire grammar, or the *rules* of the language. Grammar is about the *relationships* between people and things and their characteristics: 'who does what to whom?' 'whose is it?' 'why did he do it?' 'how did he do it?' 'where is it?' and so on. Play can help your baby and toddler to understand the relationships between things and is probably one of the ways in

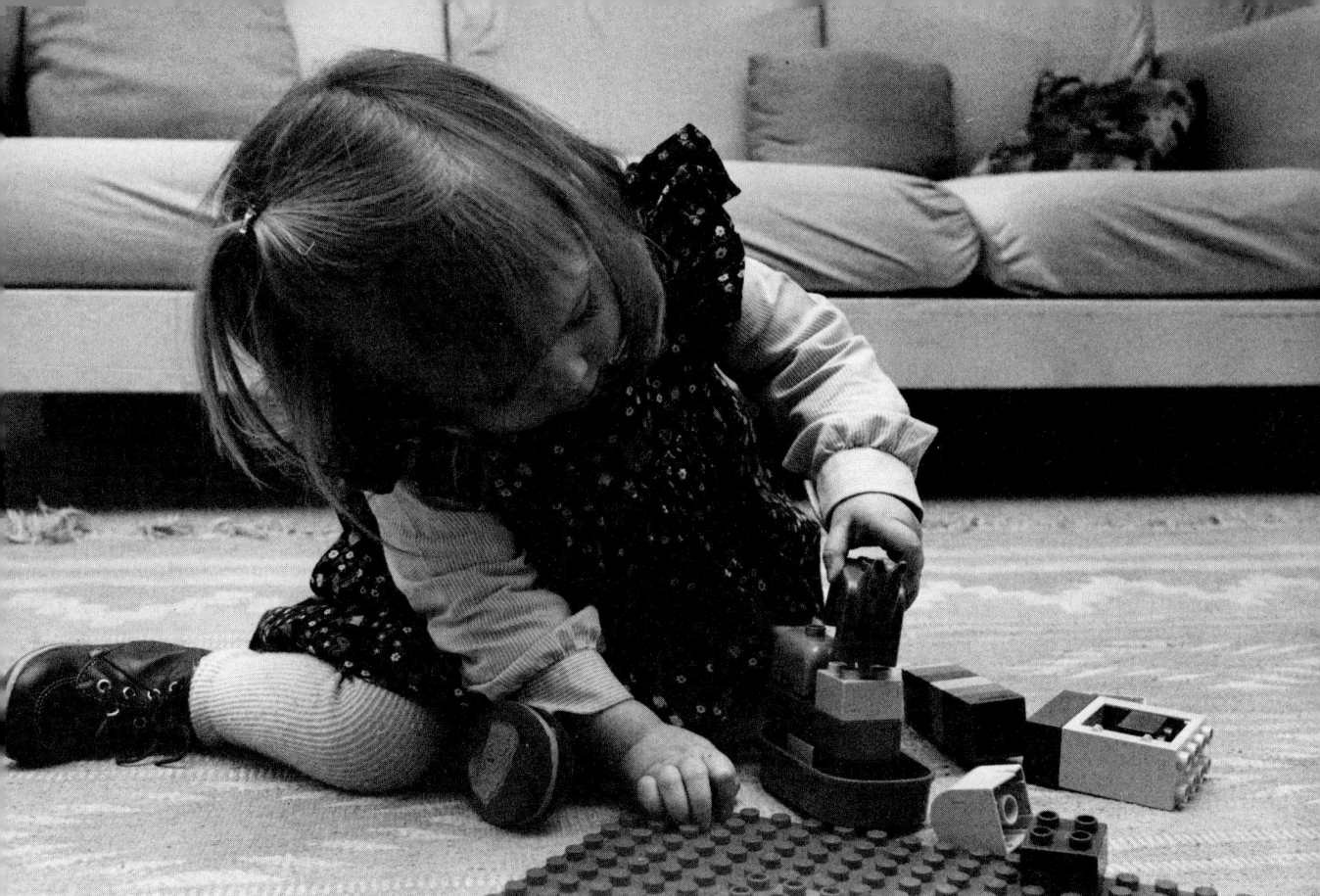

The horse rides on the boat – learning relationships between things.

which he manages to achieve the awesomely complicated task of learning the rules of his language when he is only three or four years old – years and years before he is fully matured as a human adult.

Without turning it into a tedious exercise, you can use play to encourage your baby's learning about relationships: 'The teddy kisses the doll'; 'The doll kisses the teddy'; 'The cup is *on* the table'; 'Now it's *under* the table'; 'Where's the cup?'; 'Give it to me'; 'Now give it to auntie'. You will recognise these apparently mundane examples from your own everyday conversations, of course. But perhaps you can *see* that in these mundane exchanges, accompanied by eloquent gestures (like putting your hand out) and patient repetitions when your baby doesn't get it right the first time, plus hugs and praises when he does get it right, are the foundations of the confident grammatical speech that he will be producing by the time he is four years old.

5

The First Non-Crying Sounds

'Ba ba, ma ma, ta ta . . .
gagaga . . . kekeke . . .
ajo, amawijo, popi. . . .'

Eight- to twelve-month-old baby, talking to his parents.

In the first year the baby works his way through a whole repertoire of non-crying sounds which all form part of the run-up to proper speech. These are often associated with the gestures and cries he has already learned as a way of getting attention and of communicating.

'Lèlèlèlè', cries the newborn, as if he were asking for his milk in French. You were probably prepared for his crying but you may be very surprised at how striking *silence* can be in a newborn baby. Of course your baby may lay quietly and contentedly in your arms after a feed, but on the whole, for the first few weeks of life, he will cry as soon as he wakes. It is a magical feeling when you, or an older brother or sister, lifts the crying newborn out of his cot and he stops in mid-scream, apparently anticipating food. And it can be even more magical when you peep in his crib and see he is awake and intently contemplating the ceiling or the mobile and toys you have suspended over his crib.

Soon you become aware that your baby is awake by little noises coming from the crib. As he lies there, he may gurgle and 'sing'. After six to eight weeks he starts responding with little gurgling noises to the games you play with him, or he coos delightedly in your arms or in his little chair or cot. Cooing gradually gives way to the deliberate cheerful sounds that we call babbling, often repeated syllables like 'ba', 'ta', and 'ma', and a little later 'baba', 'mamma' and 'tata'. Babbling sounds are always happy sounds. When he is cross or hungry the baby cries.

It is often thought that babbling babies produce all the sounds that are used in *every* one of the languages of the world. This is not quite true. What happens is that in the first eight months or so your baby produces the same babbling sounds as other babies of any nationality, but the range of sounds he uses is restricted to certain vowels and consonants. Initially your baby will experiment with combinations consisting of *k* and *g* followed by the vowels *a*, *o* or *e*. These consonants are soon dropped in favour of those that are produced in the front of the mouth or with the lips such as *t, d, p, m* and *b*. Babies everywhere steer well clear of *ch* sounds like the final consonant in Scottish *loch* or combinations of two or more consonants.[39]

Your baby is babbling properly when he combines single syllables like 'ba' and 'ta' into longer stretches like 'tatatata' and 'baba' with varying intonations and pauses in between. Now it sounds more and more as if he is holding conversations with you. Babies hearing a lot of speech definitely babble more, especially when alone, and if they see adults responding to their sounds with smiles and talk.[40]

In fact connecting the *sound* of you talking to him with the *sight* of you talking is extremely important to your baby. Second or later babies may hear a lot of speech directed at older siblings, but through the lack of face-to-face conversations with their mothers, they may not talk as early or as much as firstborns. One study demonstrated that babies of a few months old expected human voices to come from mouths.[41] Each baby saw his mother through a soundproof glass screen talking at him, but the sound of her voice would come from either side of the room where the babies were, or from a position straight ahead of them. The babies became bemused and slightly upset if the voice appeared to come from anywhere else than straight from their mother's mouth.

Another recent study showed that at four or five months babies relate the shape of the speaker's mouth to particular speech sounds.[42] They recognise that *a* comes from a wide open mouth and *i* from a mouth with spread lips for instance. Their ability to detect these differences will stand them in good stead when they first attempt to reproduce the sounds of their own language at around a year.

More babble and jargon

Around the middle of the first year when the babbling sequences have become longer, it will become very obvious that your baby is taking turns with you in producing sounds and listening attentively to your responses. The baby shows the same interest when conversing with an older brother or sister, even if the age gap is no more than fifteen months. The toddler's speech is a source of delight to both children. One set of girl twins held this kind of conversation with a blackbird who would come to visit them as they were out in their cots on a high-up balcony. The same twins at this stage convinced their parents that they were telling each other dubious jokes by the way one would babble while the other paused and then burst into raucous laughter.

It is not long before your baby will produce combinations of two or more syllables with different vowels in each, such as *ajo*, *amawijo*, or *popi*. This kind of baby talk is known as 'jargon'. The stretches of sound your baby produces sound more and more like true sentences. Whereas your baby frequently used *l* and *r* in babbling, these sounds now disappear altogether and he may talk about *norry* rather than *lorry* until he is almost three! In languages which use *l* and *r* such as English and Dutch, these speech sounds are among the last to be mastered by toddlers. 'Jargoning' is the immediate forerunner of real words and your baby may still indulge in this and babbling when he is already using some 'real' words. As the hearing baby moves towards reproducing the sounds of his own language, the deaf baby's babbling fades.

As your baby gets more practised in hearing the sounds of English, he loses his ear for distinctive sound contrasts that do not belong to the English language. Whereas in the first half of his first year he was able to distinguish between a sound pair like *cha* and *ka*, he will now begin to find this more difficult. A recent Canadian study[43] suggests that after one year babies have to be *taught* to recognise non-native sound contrasts, although they come into the world with the ability to distinguish between many more speech sounds than are used in the language spoken around them.

Children will continue to learn new languages relatively effortlessly by exposure until they are almost teenagers, but not all the new speech sounds will escape 'contamination' from the first language. Kate (five) and Owen (three), who are learning Dutch as a second language, produce certain Dutch sounds like the *w* with an English accent, but can easily be taught the correct pronunciation. The ability to sound totally authentic in a newly-learned language disappears when children are in their teens. Even if they master a large vocabulary and their grammar is flawless, adult second-language learners invariably retain a slightly foreign pronunciation.

Towards the end of the jargon period there is a change in the deliberate way your baby uses sound. He now shouts for attention! Your baby is beginning to use sounds with the intention of getting things done. Before, he babbled for the sake of the pleasant conversation with you, his dad and brothers and sisters and for the enjoyable sensations the sound of his own voice gave him. Now he discovers he can use sounds to manipulate his

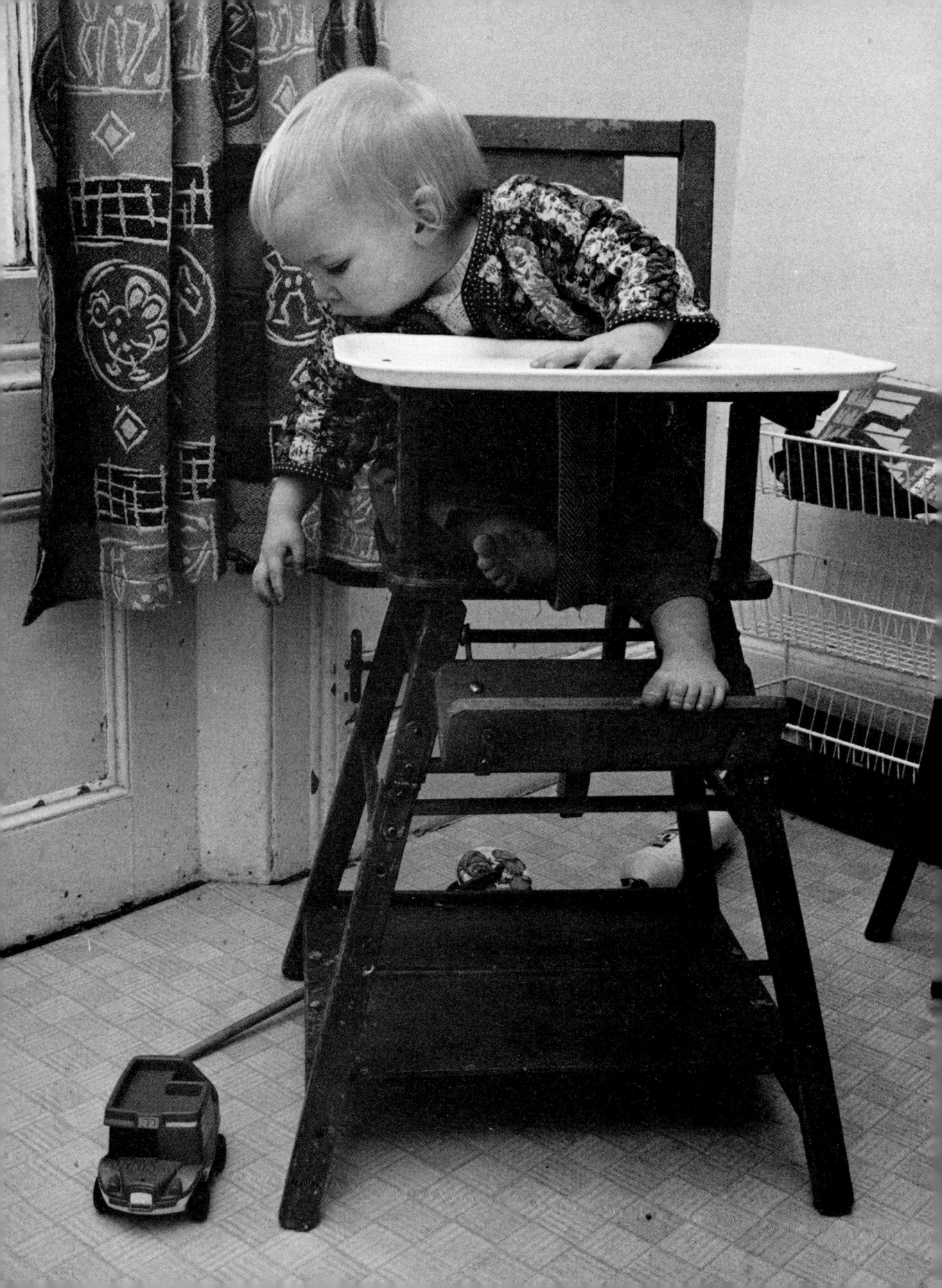

family into doing what he wants them to do: get his food, pick up the toys he dropped or simply talk directly to him rather than to each other. With the transition from intentional use of sounds for the purpose of getting attention to the deliberate use of sounds for the purpose of getting things done, your baby is on the threshold of real speech with real words.

The first year's conversational partners

In the first year your baby is most happy talking to the people most in tune with him and that means you, his father, older brothers and sisters, his nanny or childminder and if he is a twin, the other twin – all the people with whom he has forged special bonds of mutual understanding. It used to be thought that babies first became attached to their mother because she looked after them most of the time, and that other attachments developed later. It is not just the physical care you give him such as washing and feeding which determines whether your baby becomes attached to you; it is your social responsiveness, namely the interest and delight you show when he makes noises, plays and shows progress, which is responsible for this loving bond between you.

The same responsiveness in other people around him determines which other attachments your baby forms. A grandpa who gives knee-rides, sings songs and plays silly games can become a great favourite, even though your baby does not see him every day, or even every week. Twins certainly cannot look after each other in the physical sense, yet each becomes deeply attached to the other in the normal course of events.

Several developments in the second half of the first year, notably anxiety at being separated from his mother and fear of strangers, have been explained in terms of the baby's attachment to his mother, which is seen as a form of cupboard love. You supply the food and comfort which the baby fears will disappear when you go, or when a stranger takes your place. But there is a good case for thinking that, as the baby grows more competent at communicating with his mother, his fear of her leaving him becomes greater, because it will mean losing the person who *understands* him. The baby's attachments are founded on shared understanding with the people who know him well.

By seven or eight months, your baby and you, or other people he is close to, have worked out highly satisfying routines for understanding and communicating. Your baby is basking in his newfound skill of making his intentions known. He feels helpless with an adult who does not share his 'communicative code', who does not understand what he means. For him it is like being left with someone who speaks a different language. Babies left in the

Sounds have a purpose – 'please pick up my toy'.

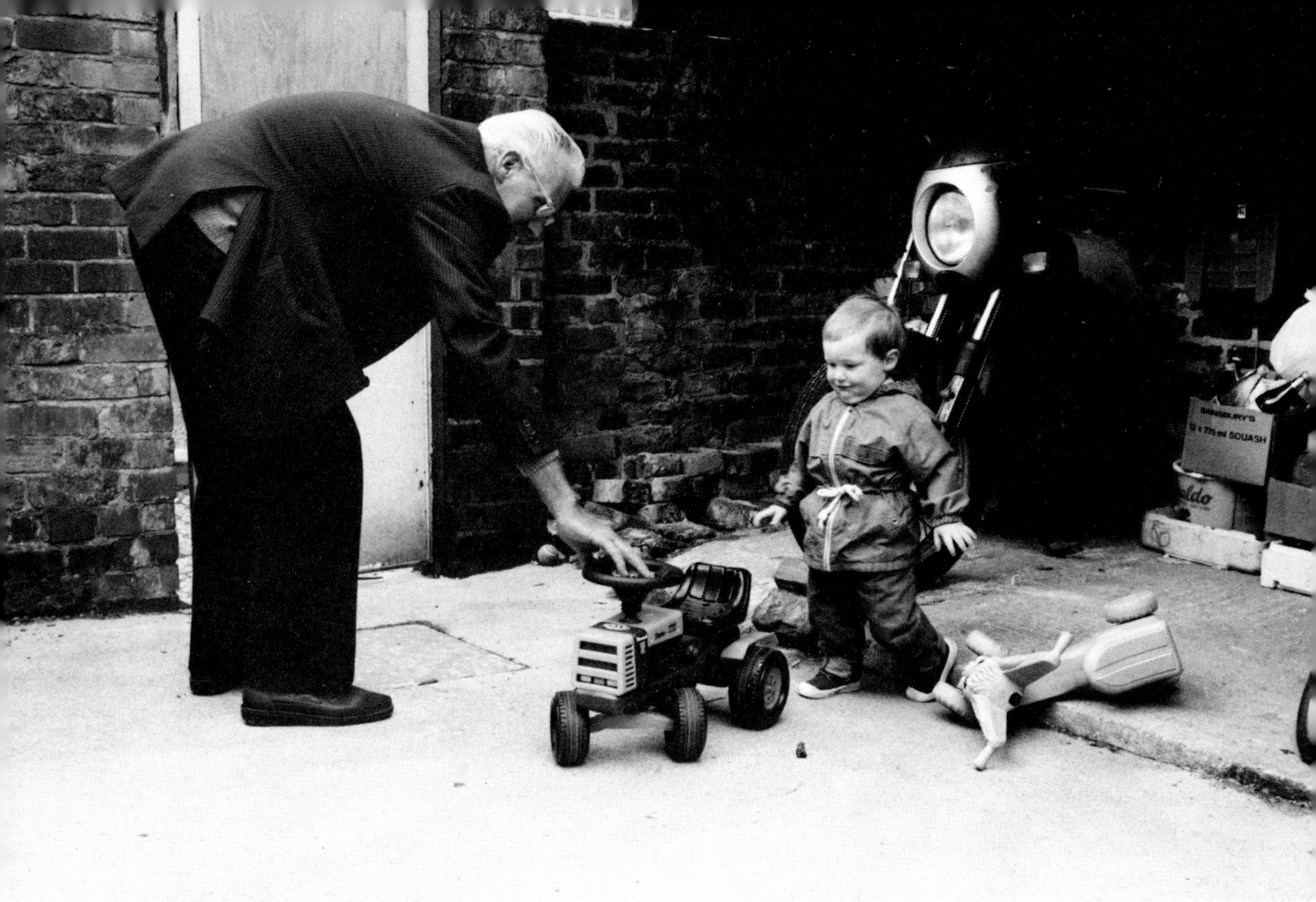

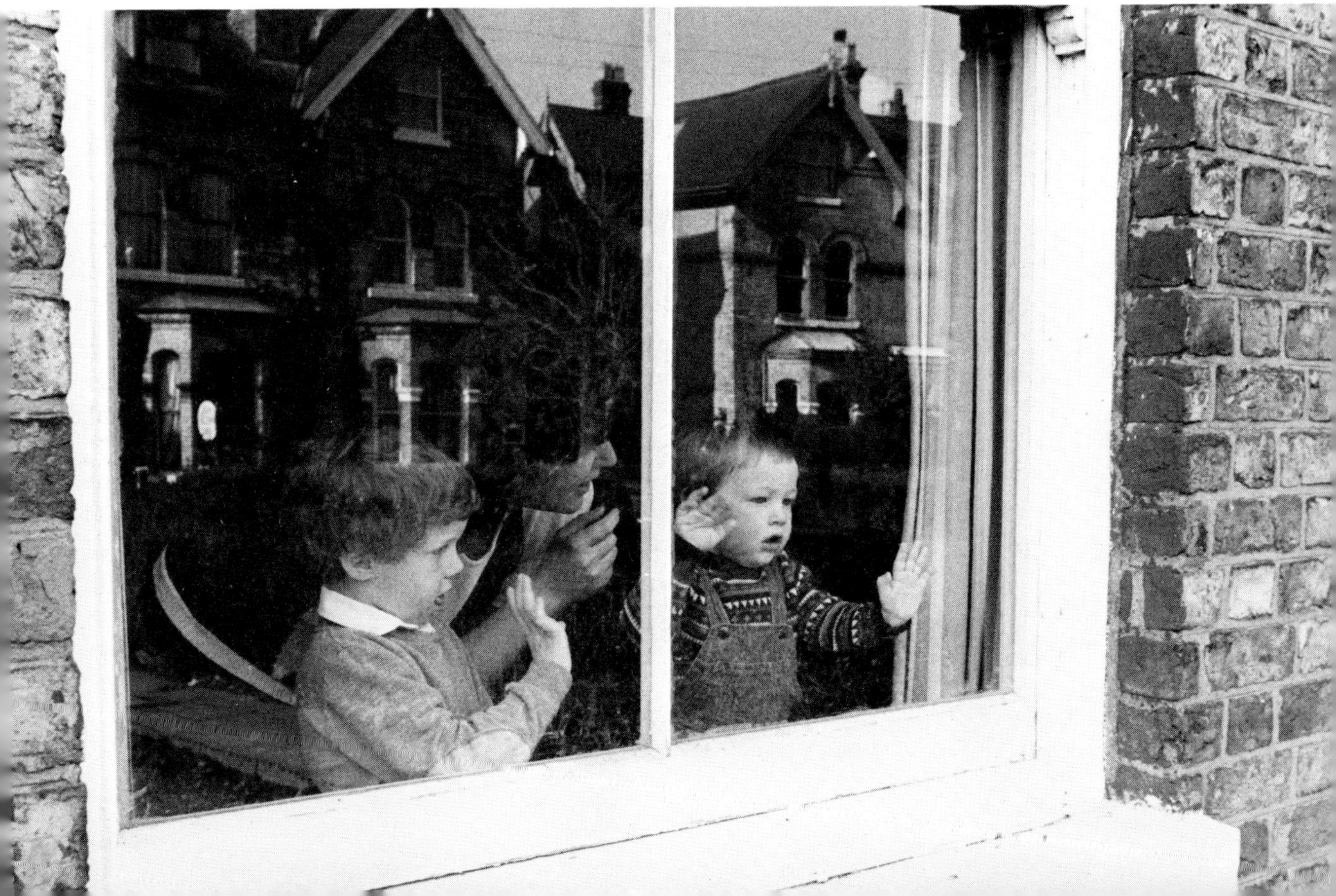

Grandfather and grandson: a special bond of mutual understanding forged in the first year.

company of older siblings or familiar adults show much less separation anxiety when their mother goes than when left in the care of relative strangers. And if your baby is used to being left for short periods with friends or relatives he knows reasonably well, he will probably not become too upset, even if there are communication problems. At least he knows that you always come back in the end!

Research in other countries indicates that separation anxiety persists longer in cultures where the mother is the main adult taking care of the baby and the babies have fewer attachments to other people who might alleviate their distress when she disappears.[44] So it is important for you to cultivate relatives and friends who share your baby's 'communicative code'. Although the term 'separation anxiety' has been used to describe the reactions of some babies to the departure of their mother, your baby may display the same behaviour when separated from his father, from his nanny or from older siblings. Also, twins often act like this when separated from each other.

Research suggests that stranger anxiety results from your baby's fear of being unable to make himself understood and does not usually show unless the stranger tries to strike up a 'conversation' with him.[45] Babies often find strangers who studiously ignore them extremely interesting to watch. From the vantage point of a familiar lap whose owner is capable of acting as an interpreter, they will happily babble at strangers or even explore their jewellery or moustaches.

As your baby becomes better able to make himself understood to less familiar people, both his fear of strangers and his separation anxiety tend to diminish. Of course personality differences between children ultimately determine how garrulous and gregarious they become, but their increasing language skills during the second year definitely herald the end of the more extreme forms of distress that can be observed in some children at about eight or nine months.

It is the way you speak to your baby and act socially towards him, that distinguishes you most clearly from other people. That gives him the confidence to explore further the use to which sounds can be put. A special name has been given to the kind of speech you direct at your baby: 'motherese'.[46] Your way of speaking to him helps to make it possible for him to communicate effectively even before his first birthday and well before the emergence of real words.

'Mother-language'

Your baby now realises goodbye does not mean farewell.

Right from the start mothers interpret all their baby's non-crying sounds as deliberate attempts at conversation and this includes coughs, yawns, sneezes and burps. You answer all vocalisations by your baby as if he were your partner in conversation and all the speech you direct at him aims to elicit a response.

Even in the first few months, mothers leave pauses for their babies to 'answer' their questions and, interestingly, direct no questions at them when they are drinking or have their mouths full. In this way your baby is introduced to one of the cornerstones of successful conversation: taking turns.[47]

This kind of conversation, which you begin immediately after your baby's birth, appears to become more satisfying, even if unconsciously so, after the first two months, when your baby smiles readily, is capable of gazing with concentration into your eyes and makes delightful little cooing and gurgling noises. At this stage the mother in rural Kenya stops talking of her baby as a 'monkey' and starts to use the word 'child' to describe him.

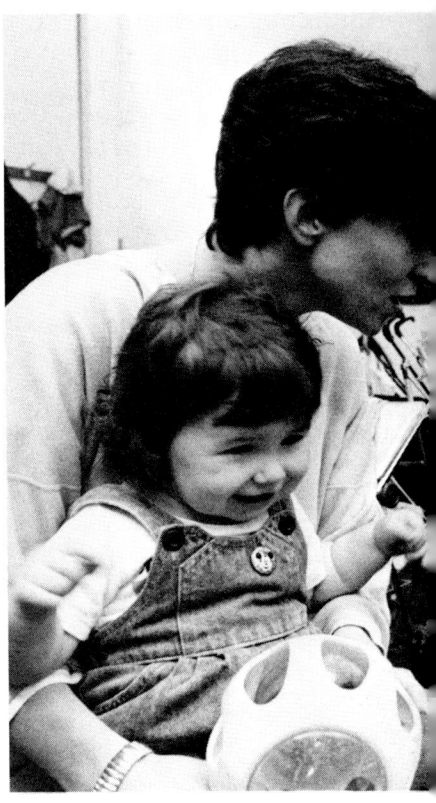

Although, as we saw, there are major changes in the sounds that your baby produces in the course of his first year, your speech as his mother changes hardly at all. At around seven months your babbling baby is able to fill in deliberately the gaps for replies that you leave him in your conversations. At this stage your baby will also initiate conversations by drawing your attention with sounds to topics he wants to 'discuss', such as trying to grab the passing cat and babbling loudly as he does so.

The structure of the language that you use in speaking to him, 'Motherese', is grammatically correct, has short sentences which are often repeated and which are simple, and lays the stress on the important 'topic' words, because its subject matter is limited to what the baby might be able to understand.[48]

Remember that it is not just the mother, who tailors her speech to her baby's level of understanding, but that it is a knack which comes naturally to fathers and older siblings as well.

But perhaps you are among those parents who have difficulty in adopting this kind of conversational style, to whom it does not come naturally. Perhaps you secretly wish your baby would become a more equal conversational partner a bit sooner. You may perhaps be a quiet person in the company of adults too. Knowing how important your talking is to your baby's development may help you to make a deliberate effort to try and see things from his perspective. You can make a point of commenting on all the things you do together with your baby, especially at meal-, bed- and bath-times. Using picture books even with very young babies will give you natural topics for simple, unforced conversations if you cannot find the inspiration in your everyday activities for extensive discussions.

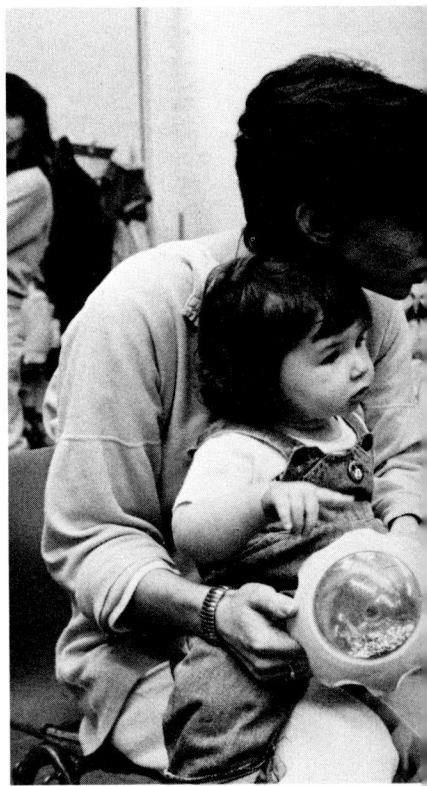

Second and later born children enjoy the advantage of a mother who has had to become used to a fairly constant conver-

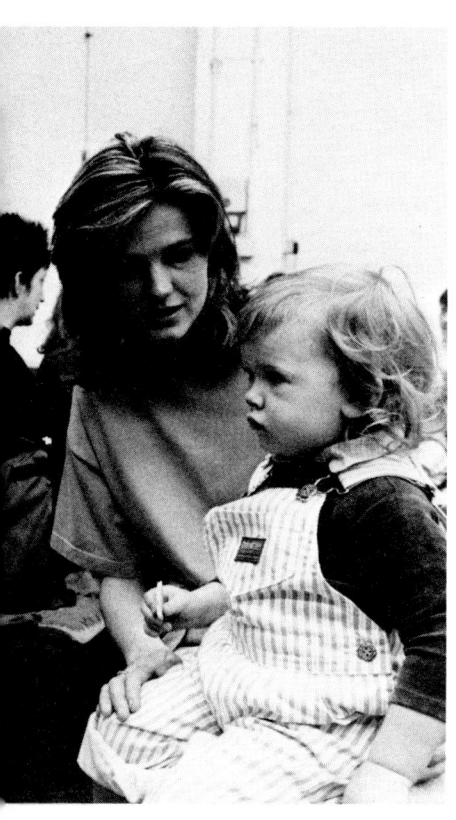
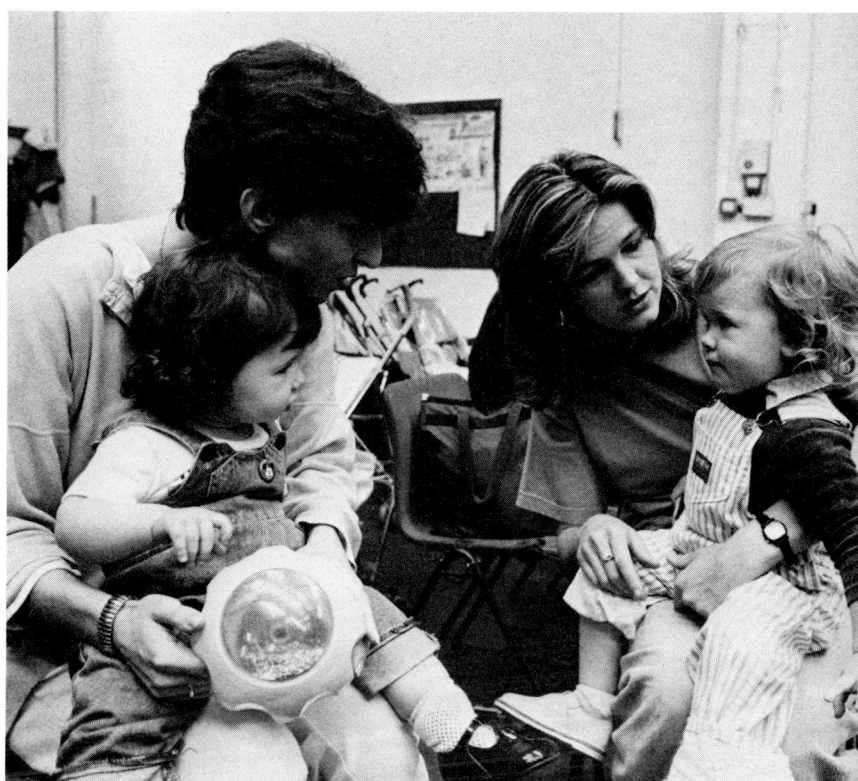
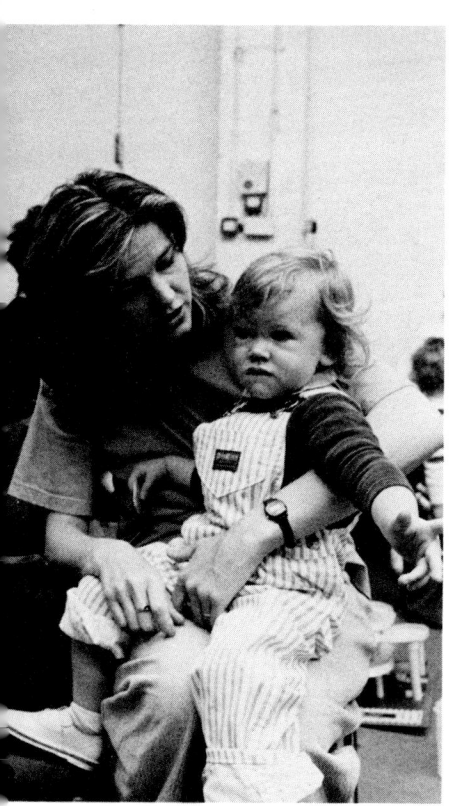
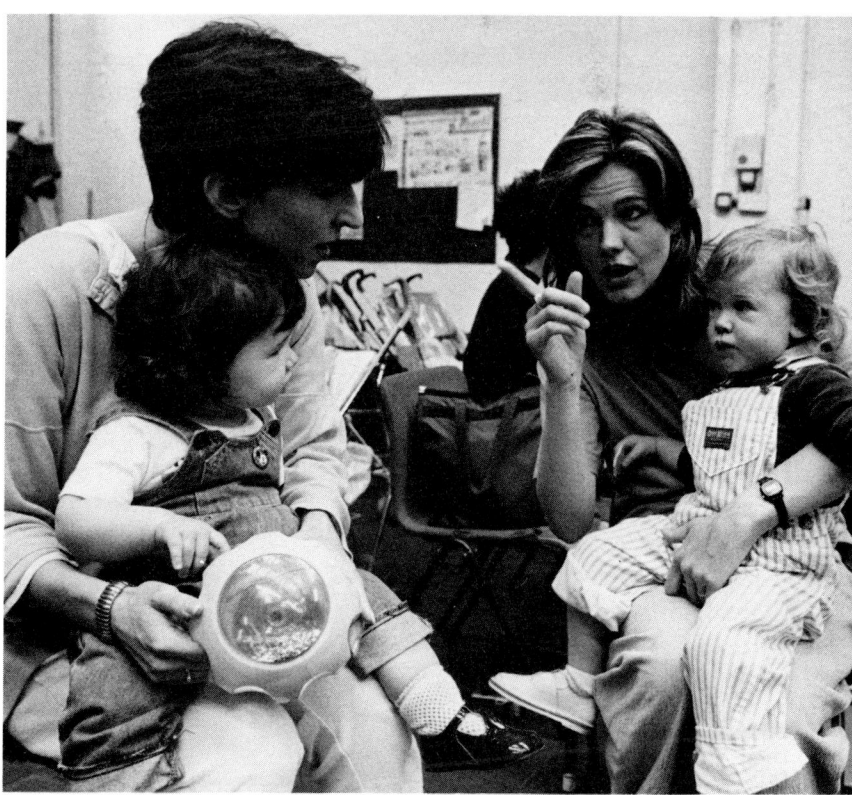

Baby and adult need to understand each other's code for communication to take place.

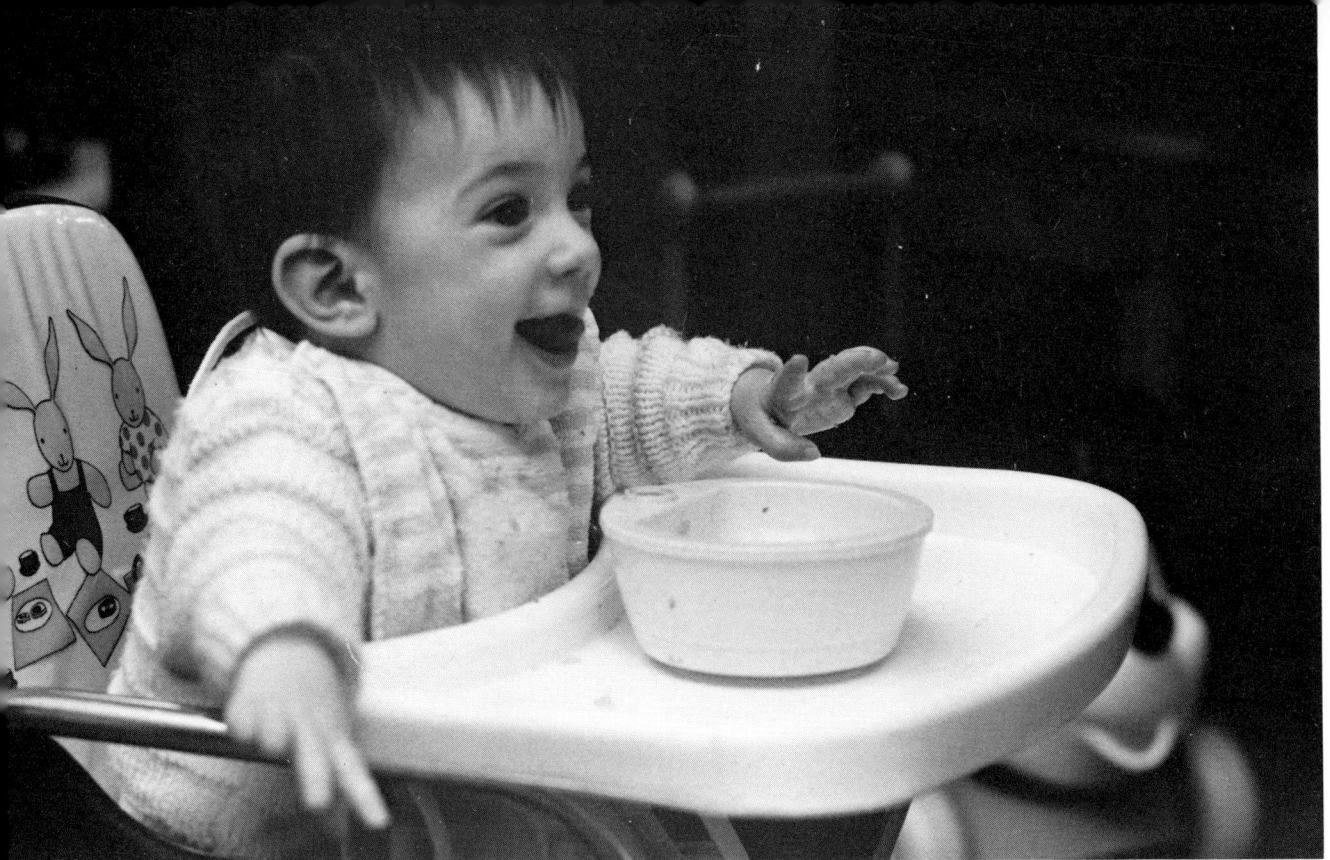

Even without words, sociable occasions like mealtimes produce lots of happy babbling.

sational exchange, for few toddlers stay silent for very long. There is normally an increased amount of conversation going on in the homes of larger families which may make the conversation with a small baby sound less stilted to mothers who are uncomfortable with this. But the second baby stands to lose out on face-to-face interaction with you, as mentioned earlier, because he must share your attention. Therefore a deliberate effort to talk to him is required from you, because the youngest member does not always manage to turn the conversation round to his chosen topic, especially in all-family conversations.

However, when the competition for attention and space to talk is at its greatest, for instance at mealtimes, babies are often at their most communicative. Spurred on by the general level of animated exchange, they happily add their shouts to the din. It is not just the general noise level that encourages vocalisations. In institutions the noise level is often quite high, but the babies there are remarkably quiet. They need to see the purpose that is served by speech in order to wish to contribute their own sounds.

If you encourage your baby by the delight you take in talking to him when he cannot yet give you a meaningful answer, you will eventually reap the rewards. The more you talk to him, the more likely he is to use his maturing speech to other members of the family and to friends without needing you as a constant interpreter, and the sooner he may feel happy and confident on his own or with you in the company of others.

6
First Words

'Mama!
Juice!
Ta.
Allgone.'

14-month-old asking for, and getting her morning refreshments, with comments.

At some time between about nine and eighteen months, your child will reach the exciting stage of producing her first single words. The first meaningful words are always *single* words; even when a child says 'allgone' or 'wassat?', she is still using these phrases as just one word. Two words together is a much more complicated development, and comes later.

A true word is quite different from the babbling that your baby has produced up to now. A true word is controlled and planned, not just a sound used in any way the child feels like. It is always used to mean the same thing, and so you know it is a word, not just playing with sounds.

What does she say?

A very common first word, much to the parents' delight, is 'mummy' or 'daddy' (usually pronounced 'mama' or 'dada'). Most first words are this kind of repeated syllable. First words always have a similar sound: they are made up of a front consonant, such as p, m, b or t (produced with the tongue at the front of the mouth), and a back vowel, such as *e* or *a* (produced with the tongue at the back). It is interesting to note that this pattern is the same, not only for English-speaking children, but for children in other parts of the world. Examples from different languages show the following: 'daddy; papa; bye-bye; mama' from English; 'dyadya (uncle); nyanya (nanny); teta (aunt)' from Russian; 'puppe (doll)' from German.[49]

The number of single words that your child learns can vary.

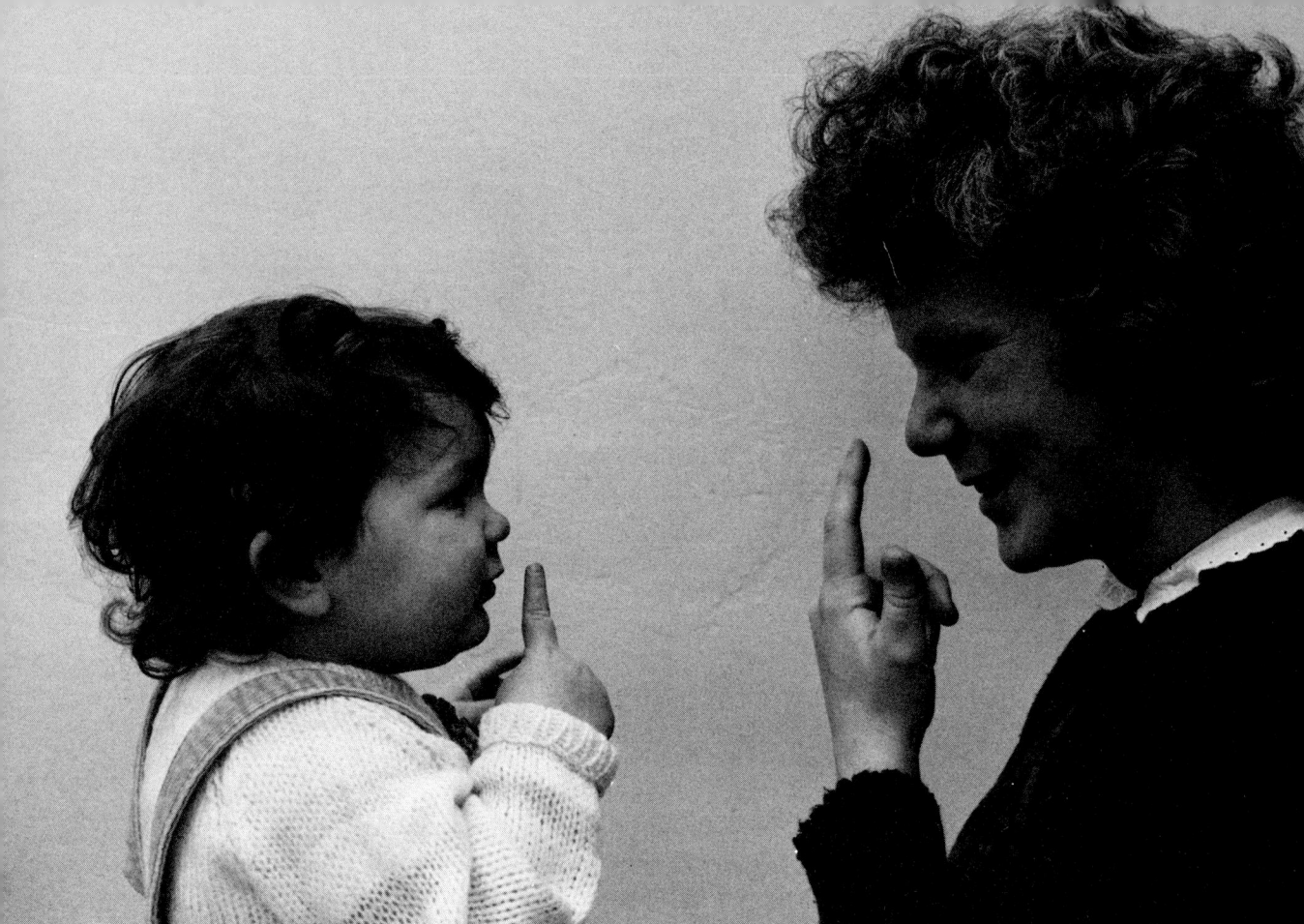

Recognising body parts: 'Yes that is my nose. Is that your nose?'.

Some children only seem to know four or five all-purpose words. Others may learn fifty words before they move on to the next stage. What your child talks about will reflect her immediate surroundings and situation. She will talk about things she has just seen or heard, not about things that happened yesterday or things that are kept upstairs. A one-word utterance can be very specific or very general; for instance 'mama' can mean just 'mother'. Or it can be a word used in lots of situations for making a request; this includes requests of people other than the real mother. (These generalised words are discussed more fully later in this chapter.)

Favourite topics

What does your child talk about most of all? Generally, children at the one-word stage talk about objects around them. Studies of children in many different countries show that children everywhere seem to agree in their choice of what is important to talk about first. A researcher who studied the first ten words of each child in a group of children found that animals, food and toys were the three categories most often referred to.[50] You might like to try making the same observations with *your* child's first ten words.

Here are some examples of the most frequently used single words:

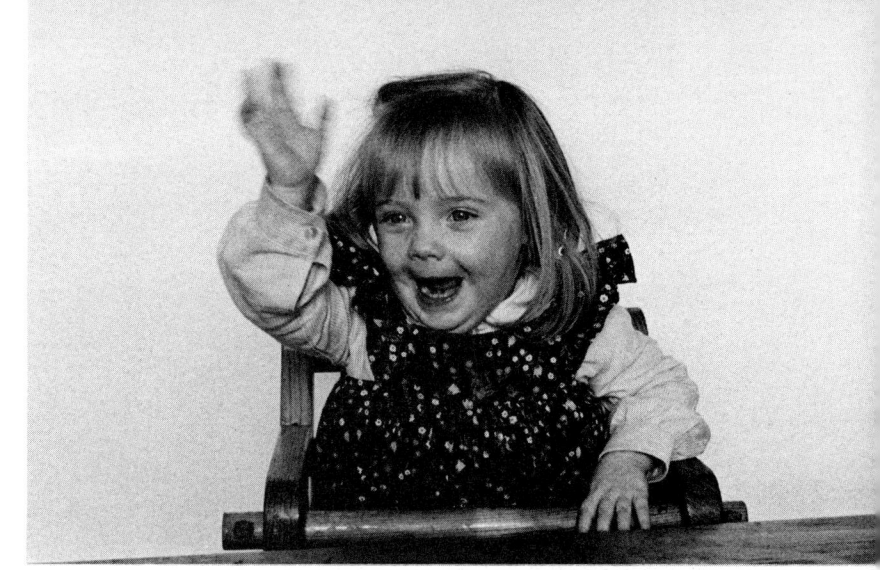

'Bye bye'

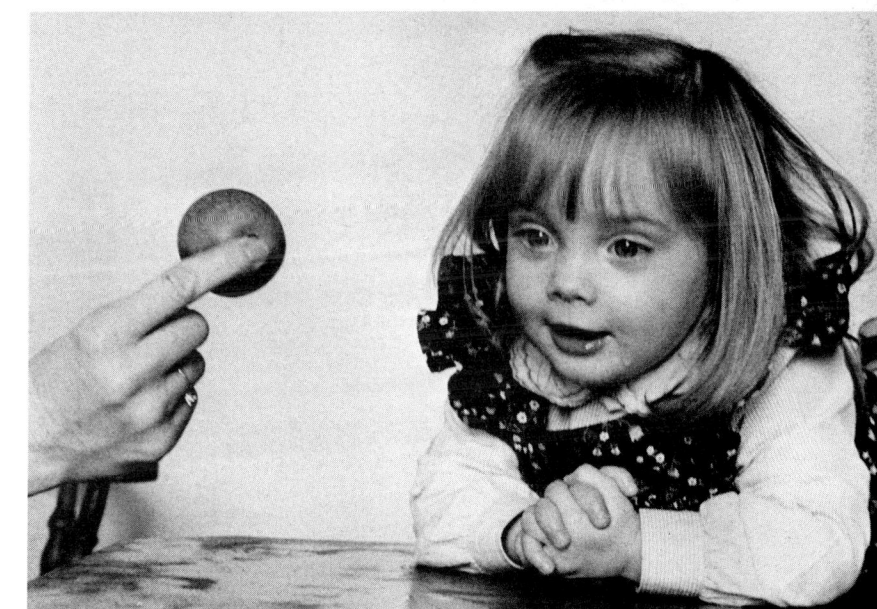

'Apple'

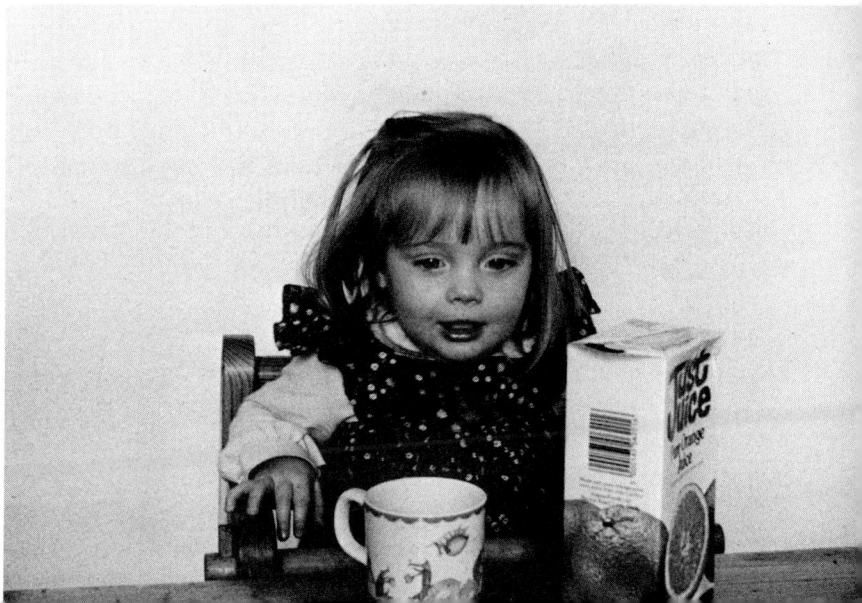

'Juice'

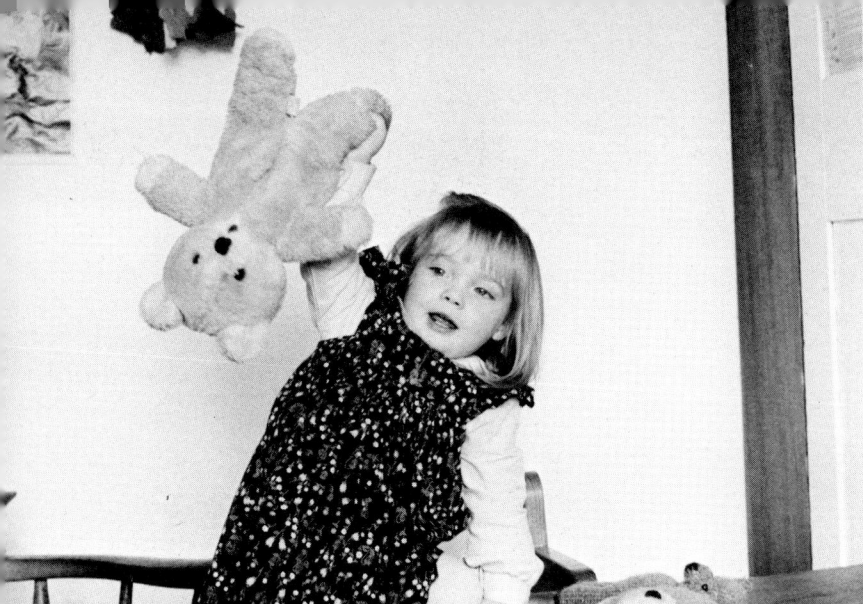

'Teddy'

'Look'

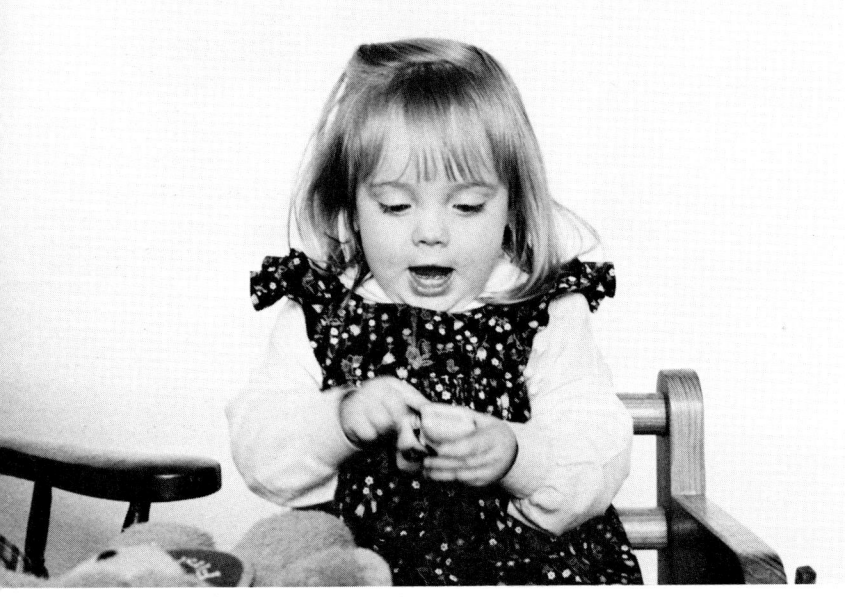

When children who have been studied reach the fifty-word stage (often many months after the first word – early words are acquired quite slowly), these are the things they talk about most often: *Food*: for example, juice, milk; *Body parts*: for example, ear, nose, eye; *Clothing*: for example, shoe, hat, sock; *Animals*: for example, dog, cat, duck; *Toys*: ball, brick, car; *People*: Mum, Dada, baby.[51]

Invented words

First words can also be words your baby has made up. For instance, Alastair used the word 'slam' for blanket. 'Slam' was a female too; Emma the teddy bear, on the other hand, was definitely male! Nicolas' first words were related to all those things he really liked; for example, 'car', 'bike', 'read', 'more', 'teddy'. He also quickly learned to position 'I' in front of these words well before he was eighteen months. James, on the other hand, was a late starter. His first words, around twenty-four months, were 'no', 'don't touch', 'bad boy', 'mummy', 'daddy' and 'Dair' (for Alastair, his older brother). Names can often be turned into special family nicknames in this way.

One-word 'sentences'

Once your child is using recognisable single words, whether her own invented ones, or obviously 'real' ones, such as 'nana' for banana, you will soon notice that she does more with them than just naming, or *labelling*, objects and people.

When looking at pictures in your lap, her excited 'nana!' tells you that she has recognised and labelled her favourite fruit. But when a few minutes later, you hear her urgent 'nana' and you see her pointing fervently at the fruit bowl, you know she is not just recognising and labelling. It is clear that your child has decided she wants to eat a banana there and then. 'Nana' formed a request: 'Can I have a banana to eat?' On yet another occasion, 'Nana' she will say with mock horror, pointing at the floor, where she has thrown it while your back was turned. You reply by echoing what she really means: 'Yes your banana has fallen on the floor. Or did you drop it?'

By using these single words, the child can make requests, she can comment on her own actions and she can describe events she sees or hears, such as her brother coming home from school. Her single words are no longer just naming things; they have become as informative as whole sentences in adult language, at least to you, and to the people who know her well.

Getting what she wants

The child has now moved beyond the 'showing off' period when she used words like 'mama' and 'dada' to the delight of her parents. She now deliberately uses words to further her goals. And she has made the important discovery that she can draw your attention to something, even when you are not watching her. No longer does she have to point; she can now guide your actions quite accurately from a distance, by shouting 'Nana!'

Naturally, it would be extremely disappointing for her now if all you did in response was to repeat her words after her, or to spend a lot of time getting her to imitate single words, such as 'hallo' or 'bye-bye'. Your child wants an appropriate response from you, and she will soon make it obvious if you misinterpret a *request* for 'nana' as a case of mere *labelling*. It is important that you do recognise it as a request; if exercising her new found skill does not

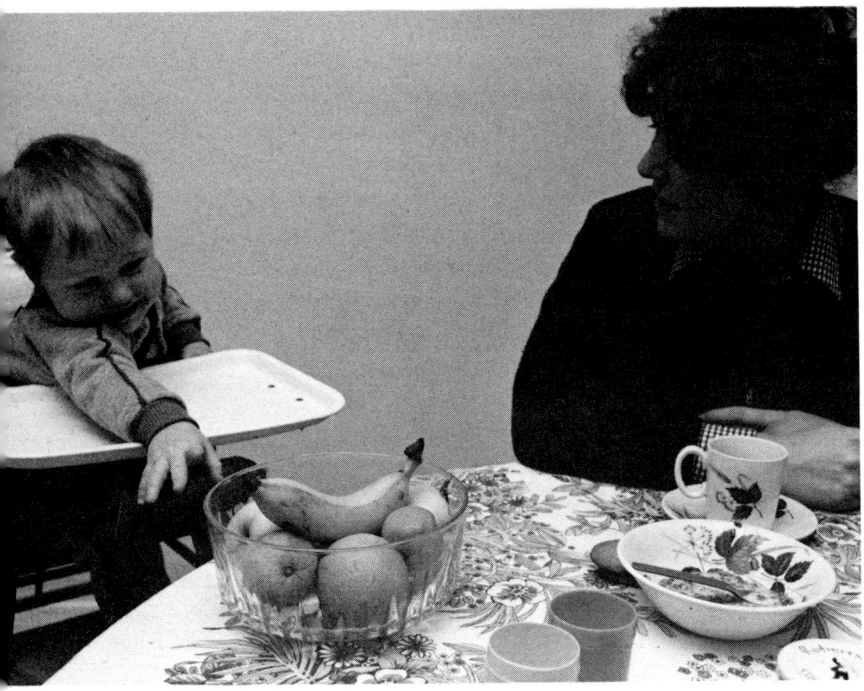

'Want that'.   'The banana?'

get her the desired banana, she might as well revert to babbling or crying for it. When you recognise her request, and act upon it, you are reinforcing her ability to use language in a useful way.

Another way of giving this reinforcement is to repeat what your child has said in your reply. Rather than saying, 'All right, I'll get you one,' you can confirm the power of the word by replying: 'You'd like a banana. Right, I'll get you a nice, big banana.' Your use of the word demonstrates that your understanding of her request came about through her speech. She now knows the word she used was necessary and appropriate because you have used it too *and* given her the banana.

Sometimes, though, she can be helped by you *misunderstanding* her. In a famous cartoon, a small girl was shown waving her hands and saying 'wawa'. The mother happily supplied her with a drink of water. The last picture showed a very puzzled child, complete with a thought-balloon which read: 'Well, now I know not to say "wawa" when I want milk.' So, sometimes, your misinterpretation can help your child to learn. So long as you read a lot into what your child says, she can learn, as in this case, about the correct and the *incorrect* use of words.

Mispronunciations

Children of this age recognise sounds which they cannot yet reproduce. So, although she says 'nana', she will understand you saying 'banana'. Indeed, if you keep saying 'nana' in imitation of

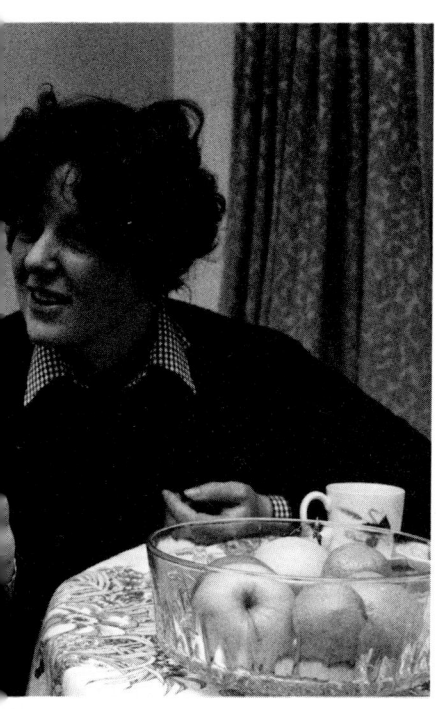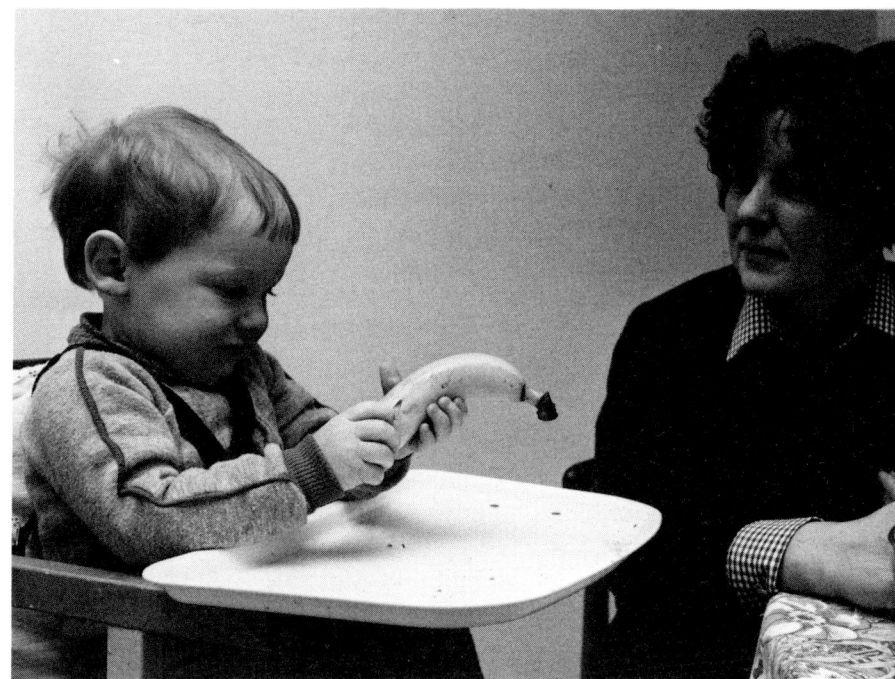

'Nana'

her, she may correct you urgently, crying 'No, nana, nana' until you say 'banana'. She cannot *say* it, but she knows what it should sound like.

Very often, too, a child of this age will use a word which does not sound like the real thing at all. For several months, one-year-old Kate talked about grapes as 'duts'. The whole family adopted this 'own' word as it helped Kate to appreciate the power of communication. In due course, she recognised that other people called her 'duts' grapes and she eventually conformed and began to say 'grapes'. When a child has an 'own' word for a special object, such as a comfort-blanket (like Alastair's 'slam'), this word may persist until the child is talking quite fluently – indeed until well past the age when the child needs a comfort blanket. Everyone in nine-year-old John's family still refers to the old bit of blanket that used to be his comforter as 'the crackie'. Your child probably has special words for things, which have become family words. Ask your friends whether their children have special words too. It might be interesting to try and work out where they came from.

Manners

When children are calling 'nana' or 'wawa' because they are hungry or thirsty, this is not the time to insist on good manners and expect a 'nana please'. The twelve-to-eighteen-month-old child is not yet ready to put two words together, let alone to observe the niceties of social behaviour. If you insist on her repeating 'please' after asking, her growing impatience at this meaningless addition may spoil the delight she takes in using speech. However, you may persuade your child to say 'ta' when you *give* her something, although it is doubtful whether she realises that this is good manners. If she has older brothers and sisters, the word 'sorry' may also make an early appearance!

Understanding

The one-word child's comprehension is already extremely sophisticated, much more so than her speech. Without thinking, you may use a long, complex sentence to your eighteen-month-old: 'Why don't you go and have a look in the brown cardboard box in the hall for some other toys to play with?' She will toddle off and do just that. Yet she herself may not be ready to string two words together for another eight months. She will use her one-word sentences to produce quite complicated requests, too, which not only you understand but also people who know her less well, such as grandparents. 'Nappy', a child of sixteen months may say, patting the relevant drawer of the chest of drawers. It means she is dirty and wants to be changed and she is reminding you of where the nappies are.

Not only nouns are employed in this way. Verbs are used similarly. 'Sit', she comments on her own action as she sits down in her little chair. 'Sit!' she says impatiently to the doll which refuses to remain propped up in the buggy. A picture of a baby in a high-chair may also produce the description: 'sit'.

Using her voice

For single-word children, intonation – or tone of voice – is also an important tool for indicating what they mean. 'Dudu' shouts a child extremely crossly and with tears in her eyes. She is trying to tell you that her sister Judy has pushed her. A word like 'deh' with a rising intonation may consistently be used to ask about objects or their names. 'Deh?' – 'what is that?' Said with a level intonation, it is meant to draw your attention to something. 'Deh!' ('Look at that!') says the child, pointing to a cat. You are fully aware that she knows the word 'cat' for cats.

'Deh?' she says, pointing at the cat sniffing around the dustbins at the front gate. She expects some kind of explanation for its presence. If all you do is confirm to her 'Yes, that is a cat', she may well repeat emphatically, 'deh! deh!', and this time, without a rising intonation. Your reply has not been sufficiently informative, she is trying to tell you. She knows that you know she can recognise a cat when she sees one. The question is, what is it doing there?

Her single words now have a greater communicative content than they had when she first started using them. She talks about the roles that objects and people fulfil, using the same words she first acquired simply to name them. 'Daddy' is the person she hears opening the door and 'daddy' indicates the owner of the dressing-gown lying on the bed. 'Nana', she says with glee on seeing a fat, yellow pencil. You intuitively know that she has not mistaken it for the real thing. 'Yes, that pencil is just like a banana,' you reply, and your child does not start yelling to be given it. She has reached another milestone; she has been making *conversation* with you.

Your contribution

Of course it takes two to make a conversation. Your side of the story is, in many ways, as important as your child's side. Your efforts at interpreting, reinforcing and explaining all help to build up your child's confidence in her increasing mastery of language.

Children do not have to be taught to talk in a formal way. Each new generation of parents is amazed at the suddenness and skill with which their young children 'come out with' new words and expressions and learn how to start, maintain and end all kinds of conversations. But this 'natural' skill does not mean that children at this early stage do not need you, and other people, to converse carefully with them. They do. Children who are not talked to or listened to very much may be slow in developing language and not so fluent when they do develop it.

Usually, situations arise quite naturally in which you have to talk to your child, and listen to her early attempts at communication. Mealtimes are an obvious time; so are walks in the pushchair, bath-times, times when she is dressed and undressed, times when she is playing, or times when you want her to do something. Only rarely will you feel the need to make *special* efforts to talk to your child and to draw her out, perhaps when she is upset and you do not know why, or when she has been visiting and you want to ask her about it.

However, if you are a busy parent, for example, a mother with a full-time job, or someone with other children, you may need to make special times for talking with your baby. A half-hour before bedtime, or getting up a bit earlier may give you the chance for some extra conversation.

How mothers talk

Studies of mothers' language to their young children show that it is quite different from the way they speak to other people. (Not only mothers adapt their speech in this way; other adults and even slightly older children, as young as four, do it.) Mothers speak simply and clearly and grammatically correctly. They use short, simple sentences and they repeat themselves a lot. They tend to ask plenty of questions and to use instructions frequently.[52] All this is partly to help the baby understand more easily and eventually to help her learn to use words more skilfully herself. But, of course, it is primarily to make your side of the conversation more effective. Conversations with toddlers *have* to include a lot of guidance, direction, explanation and questioning because that is the kind of people that toddlers are. As your child gets older, more competent and more able to express herself, your conversation to her will become less directive.

Below is an example of a mother talking to her fourteen-month-old daughter as they are sitting together while the child potters round the room, which illustrates some of the very typical ways that mothers have of talking to their 'one-word' children:

Mother: What are you holding? What's that?
Child (changing the subject): Ooh. Gar.
Mother (following child): Is that the garden? Where's the garden?
Child (changing subject again): Ker.
Mother: What's a ker? Do you mean dog? (as child points) Chair! You mean chair!
(Child rocks chair backwards and forwards and it squeaks.)
Mother: Are you rocking the chair? Are you rocking the chair?
Child (continues rocking): Ooh, ooh. (More 'jargon'.)
Mother: That's a funny noise. (Both laugh.)
Child (gesturing): Ooh?
Mother: What darling? That's the cushion.

Obviously, the mother is doing most of the talking. The child uses noises, intonations, gestures and special abbreviations ('gar', 'ker') to convey her side of the conversation. Throughout, the mother is using these to pick up clues: 'You mean chair!' and to name the chair correctly so that the little girl will eventually learn the word for herself. Nine of the mother's thirteen utterances are questions and eight of them are repetitions. Thus, she is encouraging the child to reply, to think about what she is doing and to pick up new words she might not have heard before, such as 'cushion' and 'rocking'.

The main thing is that they are both enjoying themselves. The child is playing a game with the chair and making funny noises with it. Both she and the mother are amused. Thus, this exchange is not a lesson, but a conversation. However, both parties are learning. You may have experience of similar conversations; perhaps you can think of things you and your child have learned about each other from them.

Translations

Because mothers, or special caretakers, are so 'tuned in' to their babies' conversational 'style', they often find themselves acting as interpreters for the baby to the rest of the world. This is especially important if she is left with other people; if the other people do not know that 'ker' means chair or 'duts' mean grapes, the baby can get very frustrated because no-one understands her. If she is with a childminder, nanny or babysitter, it is obviously of paramount importance that this person knows what the 'slam' or 'crackie' is, when your child is settling down to sleep!

Sometimes, though, it is another child who has to do the translating. When James, who was a slow starter, was nearly two, he made a very long, incomprehensible speech at meal time. His parents could not understand what he wanted, and when they asked him, he would not say. His brother Alastair (eighteen months older) announced that James wanted more breakfast cereal. James vigorously nodded his head, agreeing with Alastair's translation. The 'nonsense' was obviously meaningful to Alastair, who was able to translate it. But James was also able to understand Alastair's translation by nodding his head in agreement.

Second and later babies

When your first child utters her first word, this is a very exciting milestone. With a second child, you have heard it all before. Your first child may now be at the even more exciting stage of having long, complicated conversations, of making up stories and of being very creative and interesting in her use of language. In these circumstances, it can be hard for a second, or later, baby to get a look in. Twins can suffer, too, from not having very much individual conversational attention.

There is evidence to show that, the further down a family the child is, the more likely she is to be behind on language development and skills. Younger children cannot always get the attention and conversation they need in order to become confident and fluent. You may need to try harder to make times for talking with your second or later baby. Do praise her as much as you did the first when she says something.

If you kept a record of your first child's first words, do the same for the second. The comparisons might be interesting, so long as you do not criticise one for not being like the other. It is quite likely that brothers and sisters will have different conversational 'styles'.

One researcher, for example, has identified two different styles in beginning-talkers: 'referential' and 'expressive'.[50] 'Referential' implies learning about things; a child like this will use more object words and build up a larger vocabulary before she starts combining words. An 'expressive' child, on the other hand, talks more about herself and other people than about objects. She is more likely to start making two-word 'sentences' at an earlier point in her development. First children are often 'referential'; second or later children tend to be more 'expressive'. You can watch out for these kinds of differences in your own children's conversations.

One good thing for both (or all) children is to encourage the older to communicate with the younger; this is good for both their skills. When there are three, or more, of you, you have to learn to take conversational turns in threes, instead of twos. This is quite a complex social skill and it is good for children to acquire it.

7
Two Words and Beyond

Child (aged nineteen months): See dat.
Mother: Oh dear, are you losing your trousers?
Child: Trousers.
Mother: Let's pull them up.
Child: Where's potty?
Mother: Do you want the potty?
Child (confirming): Sit potty.

It is hard to realise that the conversation above with its mundane references to trousers and potties represents an exciting advance in the child's mastery of English – a big leap forwards from the one-word stage discussed in the last chapter. But it does.

Combining two words is not just a way of adding to the number of words a child can speak in a simple arithmetical way. When the child says 'Sit potty' he is not just demonstrating that he has acquired a new word, 'potty' (he had recently begun toilet training). He is also showing that the verb 'sit', which he has known for a few weeks, is something that is appropriately applied to the object, 'potty'. He also knows that the word 'potty' has to come after 'sit' because, in English, the object of the sentence has to follow the verb. If he had been referring to himself, he would have said (as he did on other occasions) 'Tony sit', because he was the subject of the sentence, the one who was doing the sitting, and in English the subject comes before the verb.

At nineteen months, this little boy has grasped the important grammatical rule of *word order*: he knows that if you change the order of words in a sentence, you change the meaning. 'Teddy sit' (Teddy sits down) is not the same as 'sit Teddy' (the doll is sitting on the teddy).

The child's other three comments in this conversation also represent advances. 'See dat' is an instruction to his mother and 'dat' (that) shows that he has learned that you do not always have to give the full name or description to something you want to draw attention to. Useful words like 'that' or 'this' or 'here', usually accompanied, in the case of toddlers this age, by pointing, tugging or other energetic gestures, successfully indicate the item under discussion. They also indicate an underlying understanding in the child that his hearer will know what he is referring to; that both share a whole body of common references, as mothers and children do by this age. If the child were talking to a complete stranger, he might say 'see trousers', if he spoke at all, because he could not be sure that the stranger would know what he was talking about if he just said 'dat'.

'Where's potty?' is almost a full sentence – only 'the' is missing. However, 'where's' at this stage is all one word to the child; he does not yet know that it is short for 'where is' and it will be quite a while before he starts using the verb 'to be' in all its many forms. Some children will say 'where potty' and not bother with the 's', and this, too, shows that they have grasped the essential part of the word to express their meaning. They want to know the location of something and 'where' is the key way of finding out. The 's' is irrelevant.

Putting words together – 'Change nappy'.

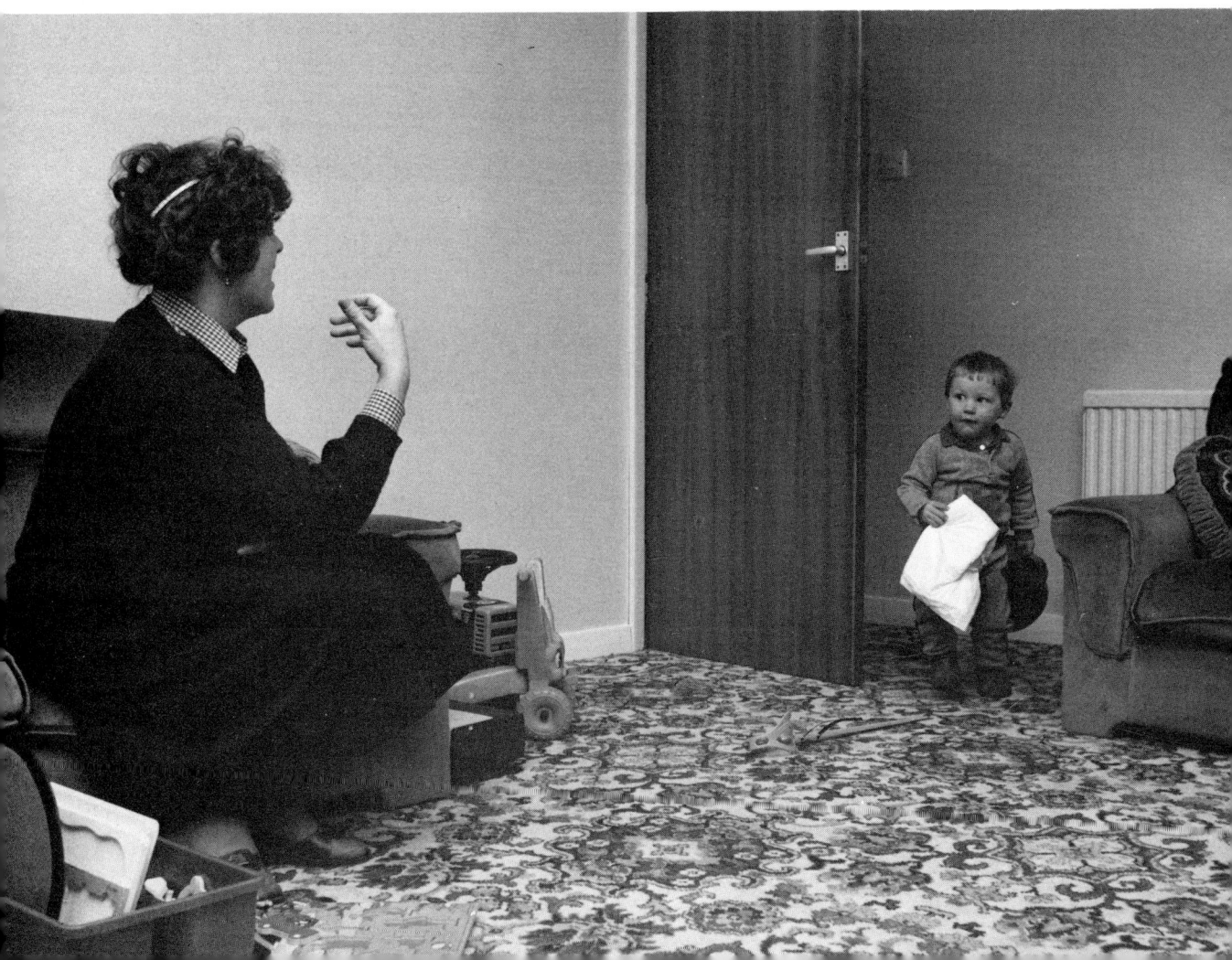

The other important advance in this particular conversation is a social rather than a linguistic one; it is a big moment in most mothers' lives when their children actually start *asking* for the potty instead of having to be led to it – another example of how language development is rooted in other important aspects of a child's development. The pleasure generated in his mother by this request may well encourage the child's confidence in his powers of linguistic expression, as well as encouraging his increasing control over bowel and bladder.

The child's other comment, 'Trousers', is back to the single-word utterance and is a bit more difficult to interpret. This particular child had a habit of repeating certain words of his mother's, perhaps to help him learn them and to practise their pronunciation. This little boy pronounced the word as 'Chousers' for quite a while. You may find your children of this age doing a lot of repeating and talking to themselves, as if they enjoyed the sounds of the words and wanted to play with them. They love the sound of new, big words and you can encourage this pleasure by telling them long words, even if you do not think they will be able to imitate them and by reading rhymes and stories to them extend their vocabulary. Hannah at two was particularly fond of the word 'soporific' which occurs in Beatrix Potter's *The Flopsy Bunnies* and quickly learned, from the context of the story, what it meant.

Sorting out one word from another

Many of the expressions used by toddlers in their second year are two words, but they are used as one word. Examples are 'wassat?', 'wanna', 'eeyare' (here you are), 'allgone' and 'doppedit' (dropped it). You will know that these expressions are seen by the child as one word because, when he *does* start combining two words, he will use the whole phrase. He will say 'doppedit bikky' or 'allgone drink' or 'eeyare Teddy' (here's the teddy). These phrases are obviously picked up all-in-one from parental comments; Hannah's mother said 'dropped it' or 'lost it' so often that Hannah attached 'it' to all kinds of words for quite some time. 'Daddy help it jump it!' she demanded when asking her father to jump her down from the table.

So how does a child know where the boundaries between words are? How does he learn to say 'dropped the bikky' and not 'droppedit bikky'? How does he realise that the word boundary comes between 'dropped' and 'it' and that these are two separate words which can be used independently? This is one of the most interesting questions of language learning and it is one for which we still do not have the full answer. It is in fact a very difficult task for a person learning a language because speech is not made up of separate and distinctly marked-off words. It is a stream of continuous sound. If you listen carefully to anyone talking you will soon realise this; and you realise it even more if you listen to someone talking a language you do not know. It is almost impossible to distinguish where one word ends and another begins. Yet small children in their first and second year of life are already learning to do this, and to do it very adeptly.

An interesting example of this ability is seen in young children's understanding of 'a' and 'the' – the articles, to give them their grammatical name. Children leave articles out in their early utterances. They get straight to the point and demand 'get cup' or 'shoe gone' or 'want lolly'. Yet they do not hear you saying 'get cup'. If you use the word 'cup' or 'lolly' or any other noun you will preface it with 'the' or 'a'. Children very rarely hear nouns without 'a' or 'the' in front of them; yet they know that these words are 'unnecessary' and that they don't 'belong' to the nouns they are always heard with. Children never say 'thecup' – they say 'cup'. They can recognise the boundary. How is still something of a mystery.

Children can recognise the function of articles well before they start to use them. (Articles come comparatively late in the sequence of grammatical rules that young children acquire in their second and third years – after the past tense, for instance.)

Some research with children of only seventeen months found that these children could understand the purpose of the article 'a'.[53] One group of children were shown a doll and told 'This is Zav', as if Zav were the doll's name. Another group were told 'This is *a* zav', as if the name 'zav' were just another type of doll, like 'model' or 'puppet'. The first group of children, who had met 'Zav', were shown some other toys like 'Zav' but they only applied the name 'Zav' to the first toy they had seen, not to the others. The second group, who had been told that the doll was '*a* zav', called all the similar dolls 'zavs'. These very young toddlers had been able to recognise that when a noun has 'a' in front of it, it is a name that can apply to whole groups of things, not a proper name like Anna or Ben, which can only apply to those individuals. This shows considerable linguistic sophistication, especially as seventeen-month-olds are not capable of using 'a' or 'the' themselves. Ingenious experiments such as this reveal the considerable knowledge of the rules of their language that young children have – something we would not know if we just considered their speech.

Although researchers are still looking at the question of *how* children work out these rules at such an early age, it does seem fairly certain that the way you speak to your child (and the way any sensitive older person speaks to him, even an older child) does give him a lot of help in clarifying the boundaries and identifying the rules. Adults speak to small children in a way that is very different from the way they speak to other adults. The way you articulate your words, slowly and clearly; your careful choice of words, using just those words that you are sure he can cope with; your tendency to use short, simple sentences, to repeat yourself and to ask questions to encourage your child to answer and to make sure he's understood: all these helpful adjustments make his task easier. Added to this is the fact that early conversational exchanges are accompanied by gestures, expressions and actions which underline the meaning, as already described. And, as mentioned too, the *topics* of first words and sentences are always familiar things, which the child can recognise and respond to, even before he knows their names. Familiarity is what enables children to acquire words that, technically, are 'difficult'; Lottie was able to identify 'puter' quite happily because a computer was a familiar item to her. A few years ago, such a word would have been incomprehensible to a one-year-old.

Two-word grammar

When a child puts two words together to make early sentences, it can have a very curt effect. These staccato sentences – 'get bikky'; 'more juice'; 'mummy kiss' – have been described as 'telegraphic', because, like telegrams, they leave all inessential words out and just use the key words that convey the most meaning. A

Learning to ask – 'Where pig?'.

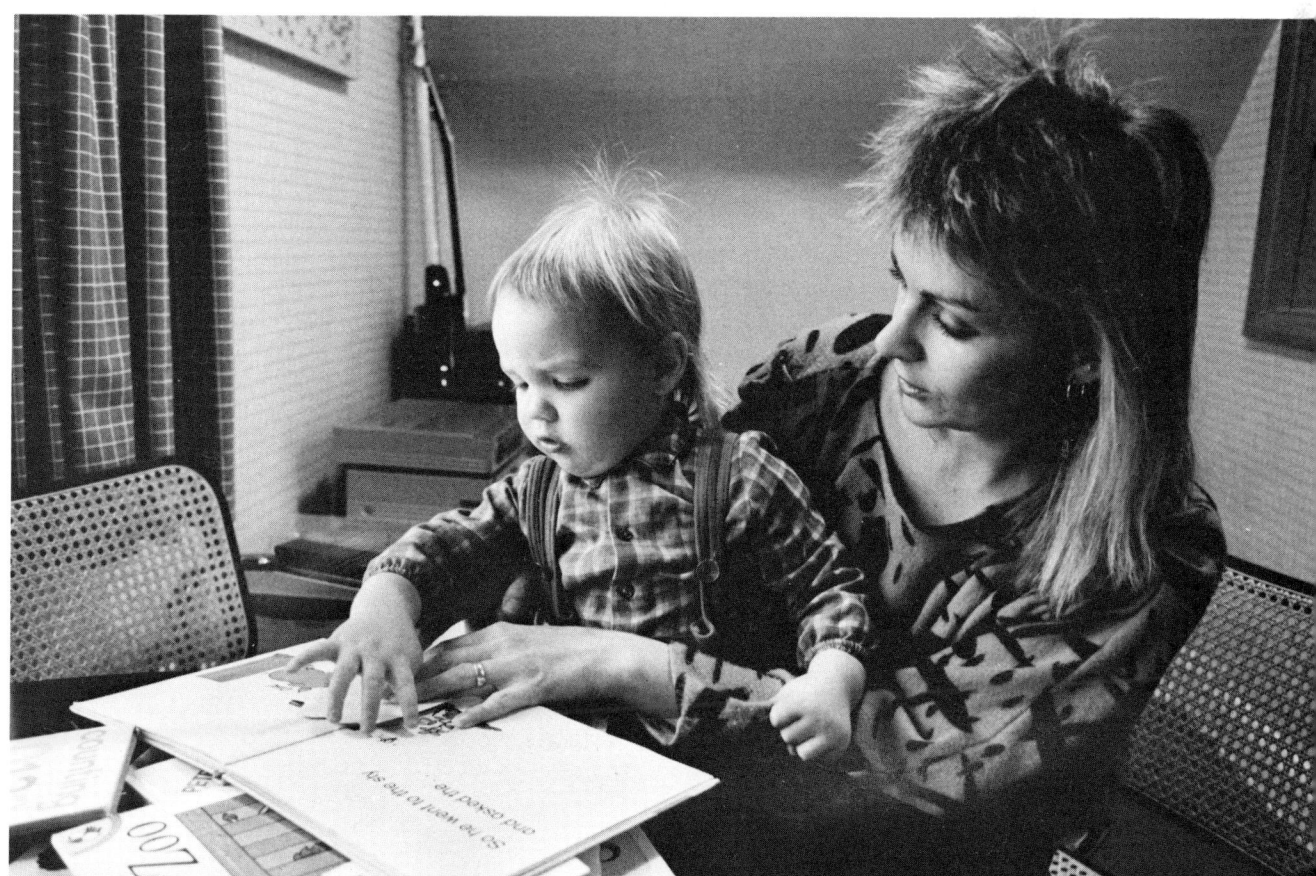

lot of such sentences, like telegrams, tend to be instructions. The rapid stream of orders issuing from a toddler beginning to use sentences no doubt contributes to the friction that arises between parents and young children at this stage. A mother can feel that she is nothing but a slave!

However, if you listen carefully, you will realise that, with just two words, a toddler can express a lot of different grammatical relationships in his first sentences. As well as getting things done, he can use them to talk *about* things, to describe, explain and point out. Using word order correctly he can say *who* did something: 'Mummy kiss' or who had something done to them: 'kiss mummy'. (He might even manage 'me kiss mummy'.)

Some of his sentences, unlike the two previous ones, will leave out the verb altogether. As grandma walks in during a mealtime, he may say, 'me dinner' (I'm eating my dinner), which is sufficiently informative for grandma, who can see what is going on. Two-word statements can effectively indicate what *belongs* to whom: 'Daddy shoe'; 'baby chair'; 'cat dish'. It is interesting to note that the small child uses the correct word order in these cases (even though he cannot yet manage the possessive 's'). He does not say, 'shoe Daddy'.

Sometimes, depending on the situation, you will interpret these statements to mean that he is telling you *where* something is. 'Baby chair' accompanied by pointing to a baby actually sitting in a chair means that the baby is *in* the chair. If the baby were not in the chair and the chair were empty, you would take 'baby chair' to mean that the chair *belonged* to the baby. Your reply to such comments – 'Yes, that is the baby's chair, but she's not in it now, is she?' – further reinforces his understanding of these distinctions in meaning. If he starts trying to drag the chair towards the baby as she sits on the floor, crying 'chair baby' (note the reversal of word order), you may guess that he is saying something like 'Let's *give* the chair to the baby'. Again, your reply will help to reinforce his understanding of the situation: 'That's very kind, but she doesn't want it now, she's playing with her toys', accompanied by an invitation to the child to join in with the play.

A very popular concept with toddlers in their second year is the concept of 'negation', or 'No', in all its many forms. Apart from using this as ways of resisting what you want him to do – 'no bath'; 'no egg'; 'no go car' – 'no' represents a widening understanding of and interest in his environment. 'No milk' or 'allgone milk' he will say in astonishment, as his cup lands on the floor and the pool of milk spreads out.

The notion of something being there, and then not there, will fascinate him, and he may deliberately spill the milk again. Children of this age get a lot of pleasure out of pouring liquid or

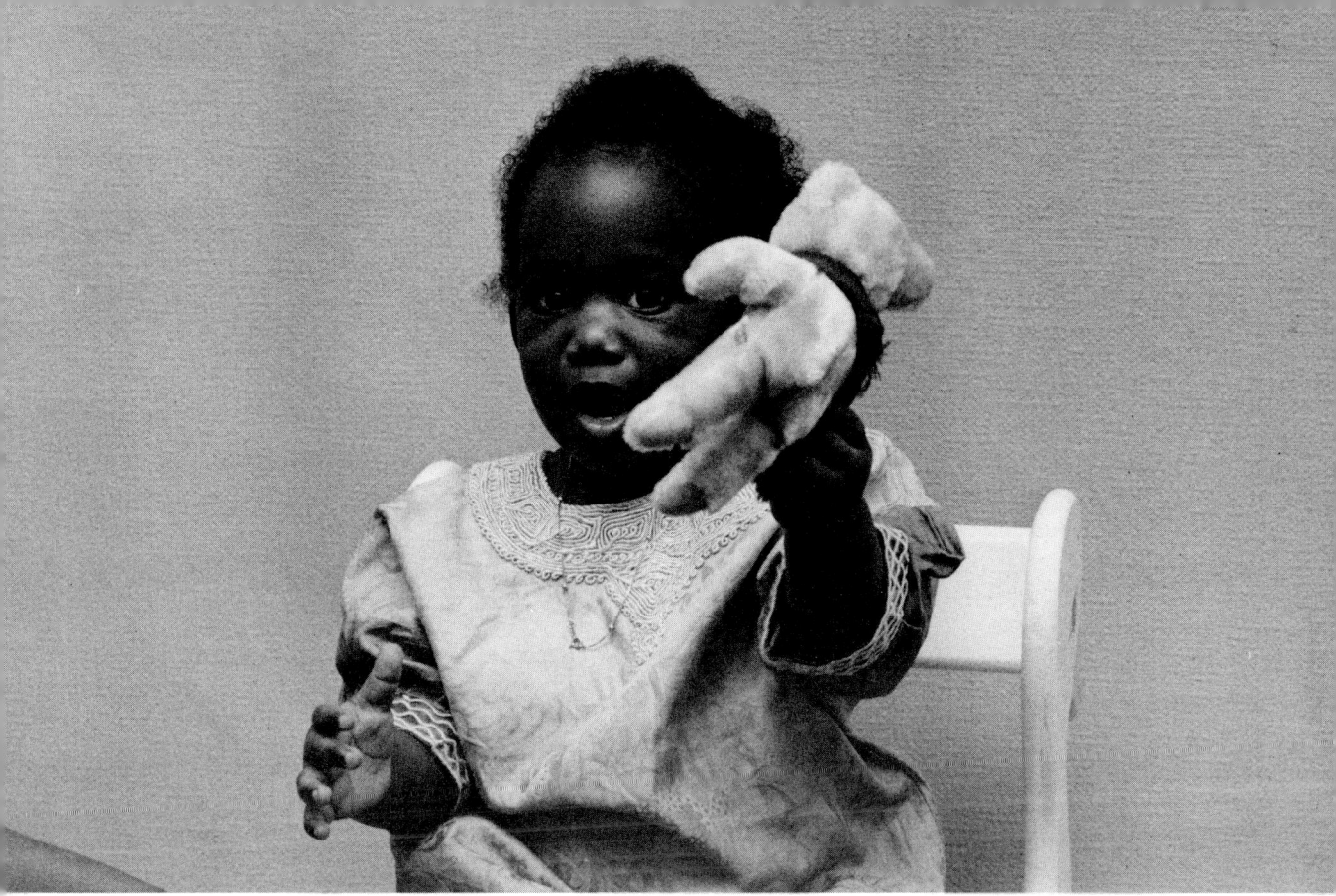

Sharing with others – 'Eeyare teddy'.

sand in and out of containers and of putting objects inside other objects. They also love taking things apart (and not putting them together again) and generally creating a chaotic mess. This can be a very trying period for you, especially when accompanied by the linguistic developments of 'no', 'can't', 'won't' that occur at this stage. But, if you can confine the chaos to particular corners of your home and particular times of the day, you can see that it is also a very exciting and important stage in your child's development.

The toddler's two-word statements can be used to point out things: 'see trousers'; 'that sticky' (that is sticky); 'daddy there'. Again, his gestures and actions will indicate to you any meaning that is not clear from the words themselves. Your response is important in reassuring him that he has the message right, or correcting him if he is not quite right: 'Daddy there? No, that's not Daddy, darling – Daddy's over here.'

During this stage, your child will also be adding to his vocabulary, picking up new and interesting nouns and verbs and useful social expressions such as 'hallo', 'goodnight', 'sorry'. His vocal expression and intonation will become more varied, which helps to make his meanings clear; rising inflections – 'Daddy there?' – will indicate to you that he is asking a question rather than making a statement. Tones of anger, amusement or exaggerated whispering – 'shhh, baby sleep' – will all help to round out what is still missing in his grammar. He will be a lot of fun to talk to and interpret at this stage, although this does demand a lot of attention and patience from you.

Once a child has reached the two-word stage and shows he has grasped the many grammatical rules that can be expressed using a simple combination of words, his speech begins to 'take off'. After taking several months to build up a list of single words and then to start tentatively combining them, the rate of acquiring new rules and combinations suddenly accelerates. By three, most children are speaking fluently and creatively and making very few grammatical mistakes. The ones they do make are usually logical, like 'taked' or 'eated'. But, even at two, many children have managed to grasp most of the essentials of producing intelligible English.

The little boy quoted at the beginning of the chapter was recorded again six months later, when he had just turned two. He

Conversations at bathtime – 'Have you lost the soap?'.

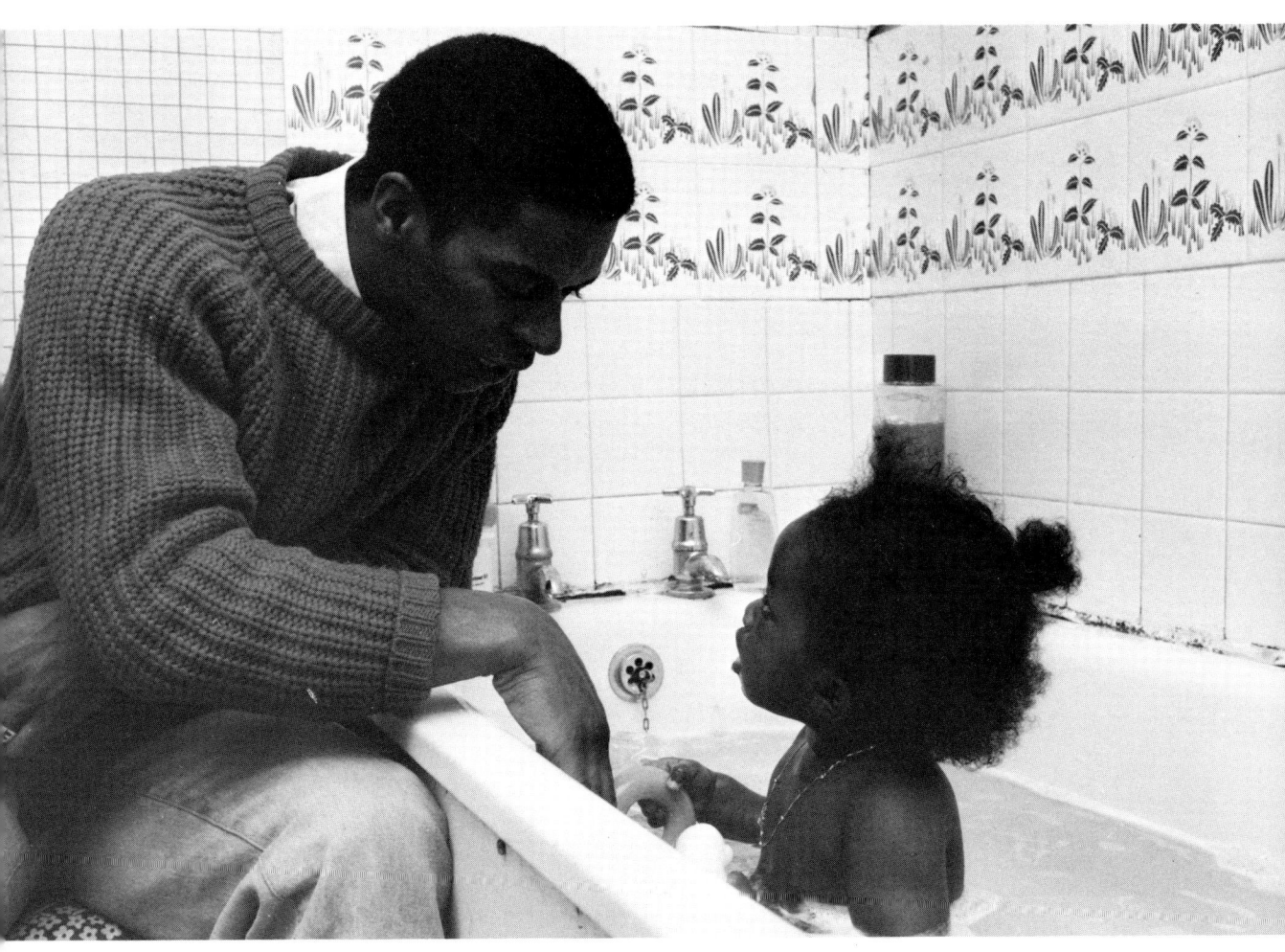

was in the bath and his mother called to him: 'Are you warm enough in there?'

Child: I are.

Mother: What are you doing?

Child: I'm cleaning the bath.

This conversation is very much more complex than the earlier one. In the first place, the child has effortlessly understood what his mother is saying to him without her being in the room. He answers her by using the correct personal pronoun 'I' (earlier he tended to use 'me') and the verb 'to be' as a description of how he is feeling (short for 'I are warm'). He has not got the form of the verb quite right yet (obviously it should be 'am'), but he has got the grammatical construction right. Then he recognises the form of his mother's question; she is asking what he is doing now, at this moment, so he recognises that he has to answer in the same vein by putting the progressive 'ing' on the end of the verb: 'I'm cleaning'.

Again, he uses the correct personal pronoun and this time, interestingly, he does not say 'I are' – he says 'I'm', short for 'I am'. He seems to be at a transitional stage, where he has nearly sorted out the different forms and uses of the verb 'to be' but has not quite got there. Obviously, his word order is correct, with subject-verb-object all where they should be in the sentence, and he uses the definite article 'the' quite automatically. No longer does he say 'clean bath'. In just this very short snatch of conversation, we can see that the child has made a huge leap in his use of the rules of his language, and in the rules of conversation with another person too. He is now a confident and successful verbal communicator.

8
The Wider World of Language

Elinor (aged thirteen months): Oh, dee dah, dee dah, dee dah. Baba baba.
Huw (aged five): That's 'Baa baa black sheep' she's singing. (singing) 'Baa baa black sheep have you any wool?'
Elinor (singing): Dee dah dee dah
Huw (joining in): Dee dah dee dah
Elinor: Ba ba ba ba ba ba ba ba ba ba
Huw: Ba ba ba ba berlaba berlaba
Together: Ba ba berlaba dee dah and so on.

Right from birth, babies are exposed to many sources of information and meaning. Discussions and studies of language development often focus almost entirely on what goes on between the baby and her mother, perhaps because it is easier to study just two people in a fairly controlled and static situation.

But, of course, even for a new baby, life is far from being controlled and static. It is full of unexpected and complex events and many people and influences surround the growing baby not just one mother. The example of 'conversation' above does not look very meaningful in cold print. But it does indicate the importance of other people, such as brothers and sisters, and of cultural influences such as songs and nursery rhymes, in the world of meanings surrounding the developing baby.

Brothers and sisters

The way a brother or sister affects your baby's language development is obviously going to be very different from the way that you do. Parents are very sensitive to their babies' behaviour and very quick to interpret it and take it further. You know how important 'the first word' is; it is a big milestone for all parents. A child will be much less worried about the baby making *progress*; his concern will be for the baby here and now and, of course, for the ways in which the baby may affect *his* life (not always for the better, he may fear).

This does not mean that young children cannot be sensitive to or understand the needs of their baby brothers and sisters. Because they are children themselves, they may be more sensitive than you are, particularly when it comes to needs and feelings. If you have more than one child, you may have noticed the occasions when the older one has heard the younger babbling or seen the baby gesturing and has said to you: 'She wants to get out of the high chair,' or 'She's hungry' or 'She wants her teddy.' If you do as the older child says, you find that he was indeed right: the baby is happy. The older child thus acts as an interpreter for the younger one.

Seeing the other's point of view

One of the most important skills in holding a conversation and in speaking at all is having some idea of the other person's point of view. Knowing the other person's opinions, state of mind, linguistic fluency, personality characteristics and so on, all make it easier to communicate with her. Language is communication and we need to have some idea of who the receiver of the message is and how she is likely to feel about it, before we say something to her.

This is a skill that a baby has to learn. Before she can utter that magic first 'bikky' or 'nana', she has to know that 'bikky' and 'nana' are sound-signals that will be recognised by the person from whom she is demanding them. She also has to have a pretty shrewd idea that the person will deliver the goods – that mother or father or nanny or brother know where bikkies and nanas are to be found and will produce one when instructed to do so.

Some theories of child development suggest that very young children cannot see another person's point of view; young children are supposed to be 'egocentric' or self-centred and thus lacking in the really sensitive skills that are needed for two-way communication. However, studies of young children together, particularly brothers and sisters, show that being with another child can greatly develop the skills of knowing how another person feels. And where the other child is a member of the same family, there is a whole shared world of objects and experiences that enable the siblings to understand each other and even to exclude the adults.

In a study of forty families having a second baby, Judy Dunn and Carol Kendrick in Cambridge found many examples of the older child showing awareness of the younger child's feelings or meanings.[54] Often, of course, the older child was expressing feelings that he would have had himself in the same situation: 'The baby wants a biscuit' can often mean that 'I, too, would like a biscuit'. But in many cases it was quite clear that the older child (in

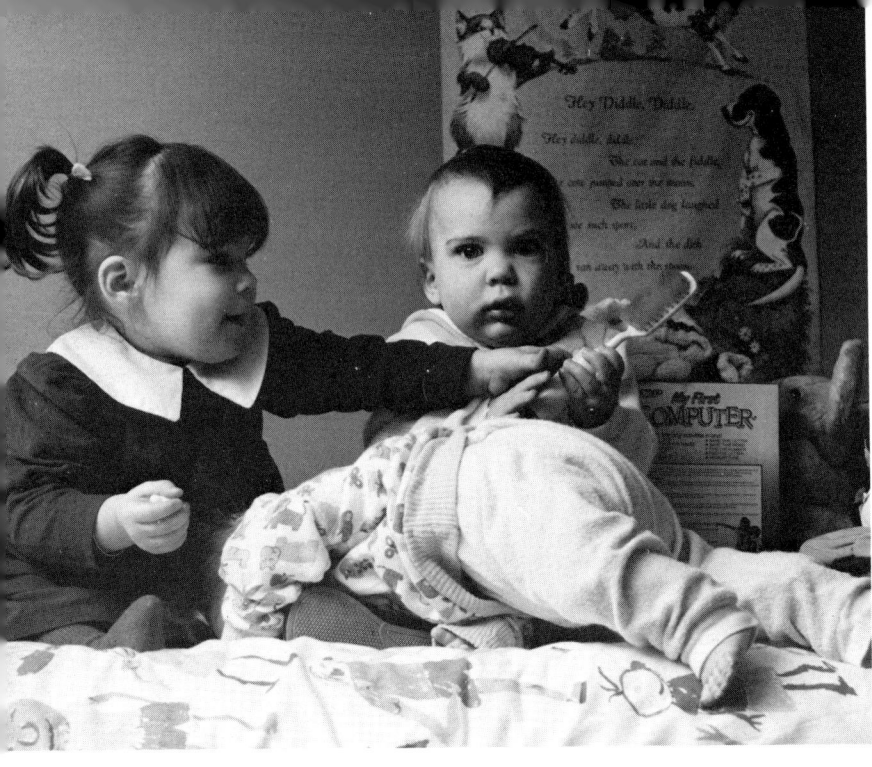
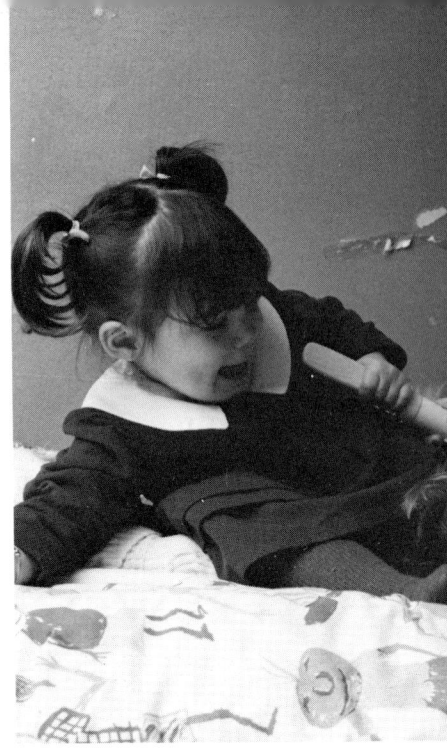

Why does baby brother always want what I've got? Siblings often fight over possessions – but still end up side by side in the end.

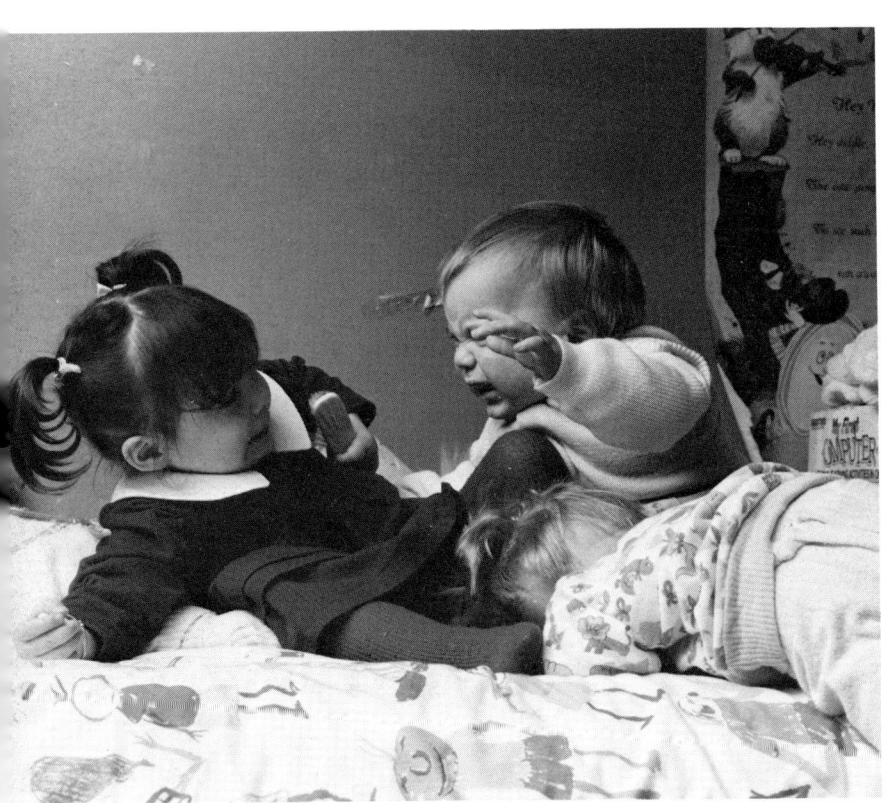
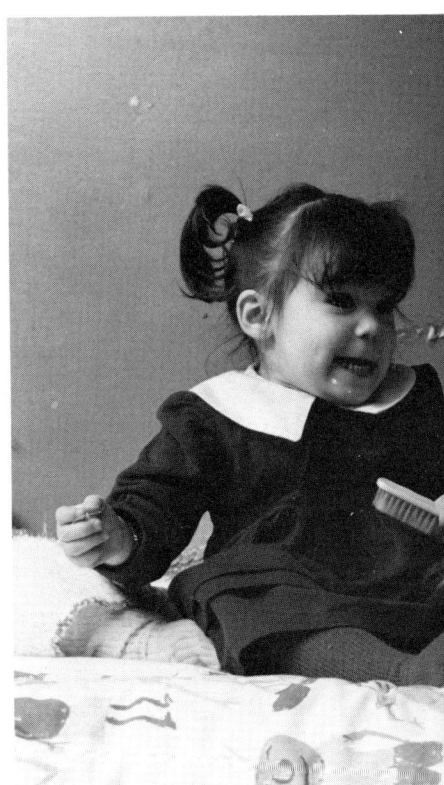

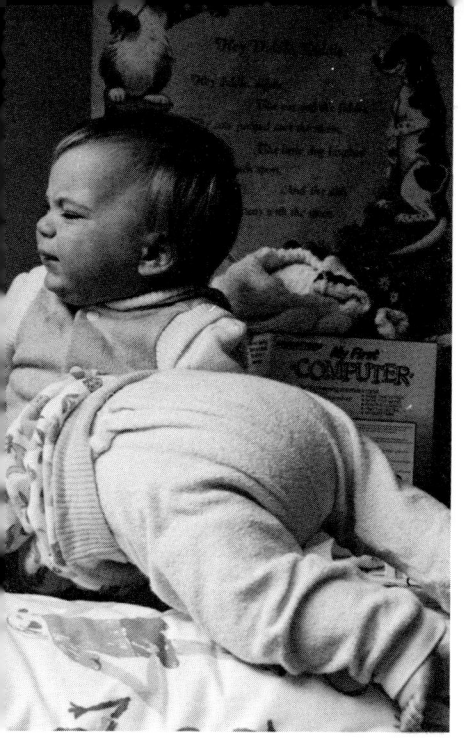
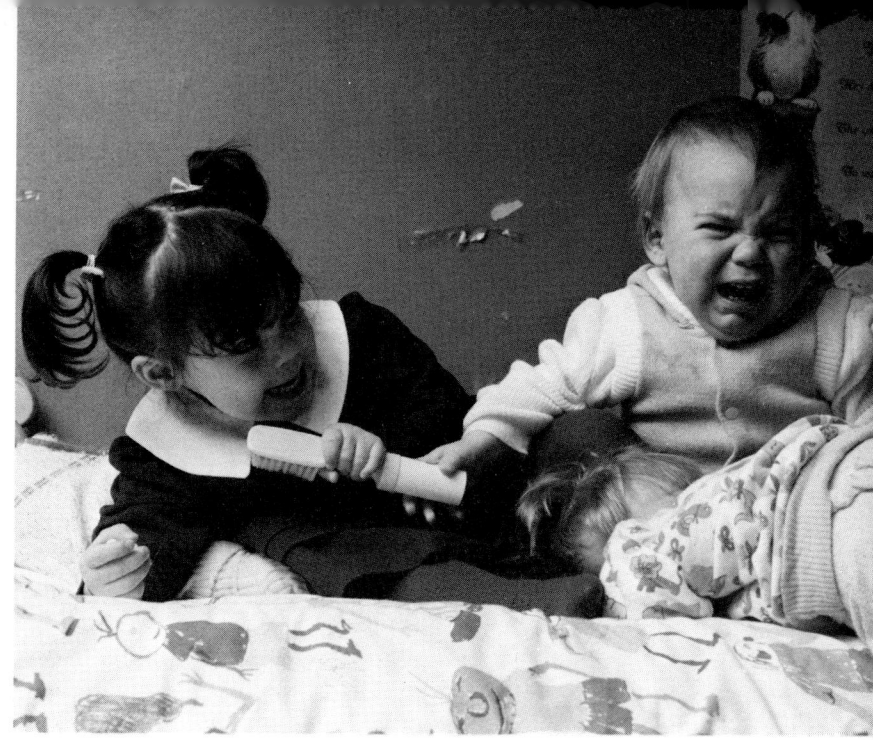
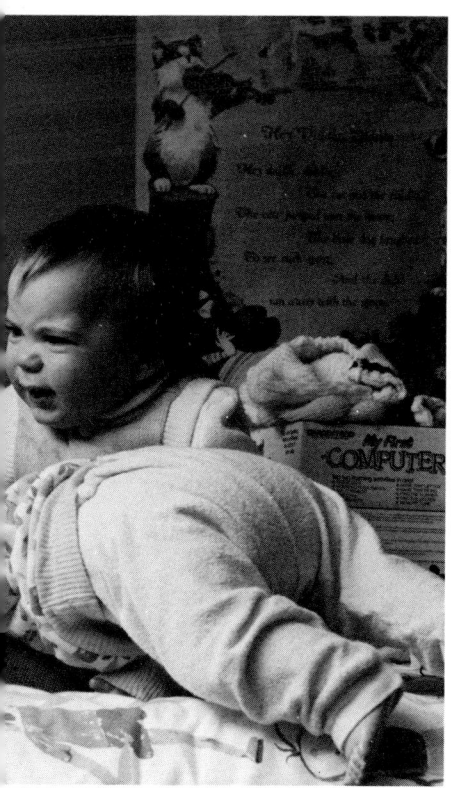
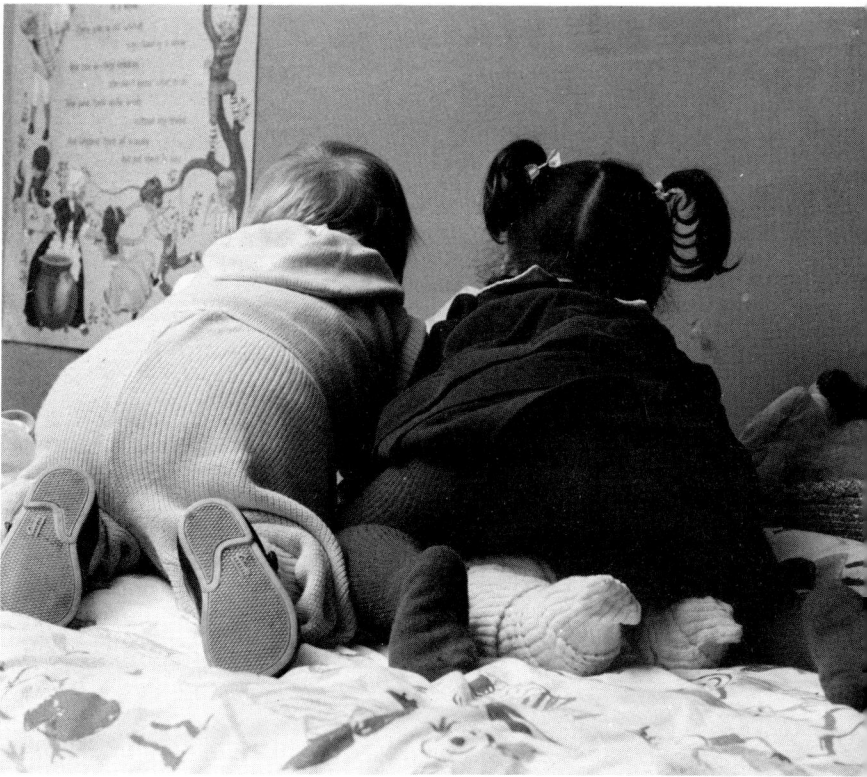

97

this study, usually around two to three years old) was able to distinguish between his own feelings and the immature baby's rather different ones. One example was of a boy who knew that the balloon his baby brother was playing with was about to pop. The older child expressed concern that the baby would be frightened by the bang and would cry. He was not so concerned about the balloon popping on his own behalf. These researchers studied the families over an extended period (from just before the second child's birth until this child was fourteen months old) and found that the number of incidents where the older child showed awareness of the second child's feelings increased over time and also became more sophisticated.

Even more interesting from our point of view was the fact that, by fourteen months, the *younger* children had begun to show awareness of the older child's feelings. Not only would they attempt to comfort an older brother or sister when they sensed they were upset, they also developed a shrewd knowledge of how to get on the older child's nerves when they wanted to. One younger child knew exactly which was the older child's favourite toy and deliberately took it. It does seem from this kind of evidence that brothers and sisters get plenty of opportunities to observe, learn about and exploit the feelings and attitudes of another person similar to themselves and this can facilitate their powers of communication, even though this is not, as yet, directly expressed in verbal language.

However, verbal skills may be encouraged by an older brother or sister too. We have already described how three-and-a-half-year-old Alastair could translate two-year-old James's 'jargon' into a request for breakfast cereal, and how James was able to understand the translation. In the example quoted at the beginning of the chapter, Huw picked up his baby sister's 'baba' and turned it into 'Baa baa black sheep', which in turn encouraged a lively singing session between them. Brothers and sisters can build up a stock of shared words, expressions, gestures and games which enable them to communicate with each other very effectively and which may have *you* completely baffled. You may find it interesting to observe your children's behaviour together and notice the occasions when each seems to be interpreting the other's behaviour or sounds. Even if your little one is not yet producing any speech, if she is able to understand what her older sibling does and is able to co-operate with him, if he makes her laugh (or cry) or if she can do the same to him, then you can be confident that she is developing her powers of communication just the same.

Brothers and sisters can understand each other's language well, and teach and learn from each other.

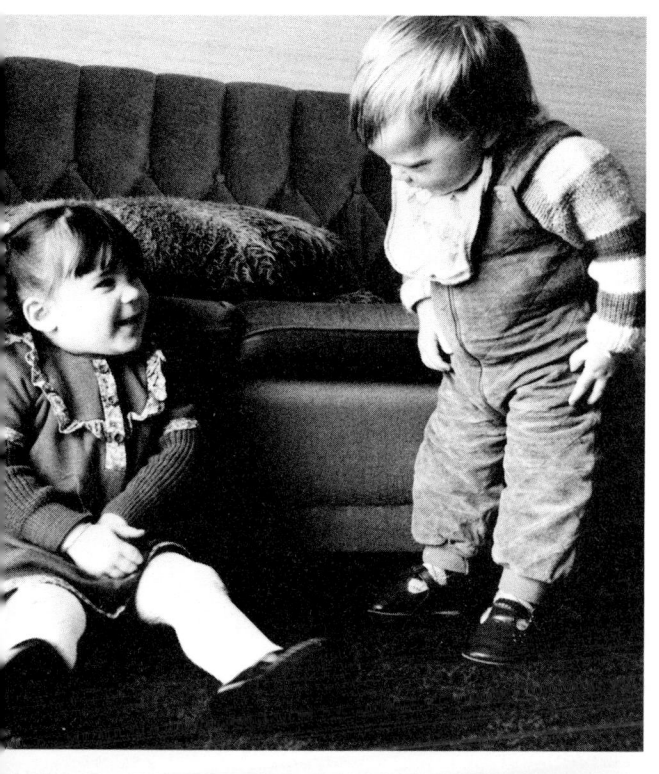
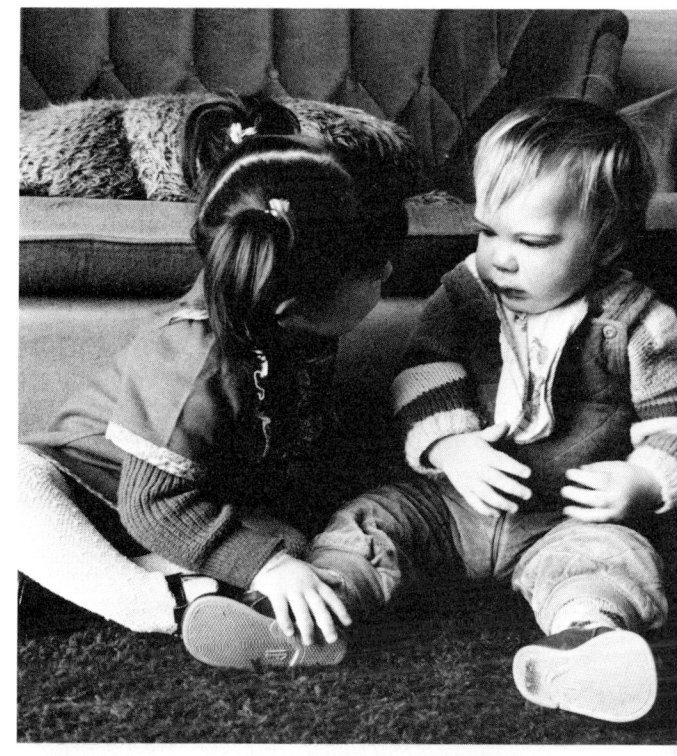
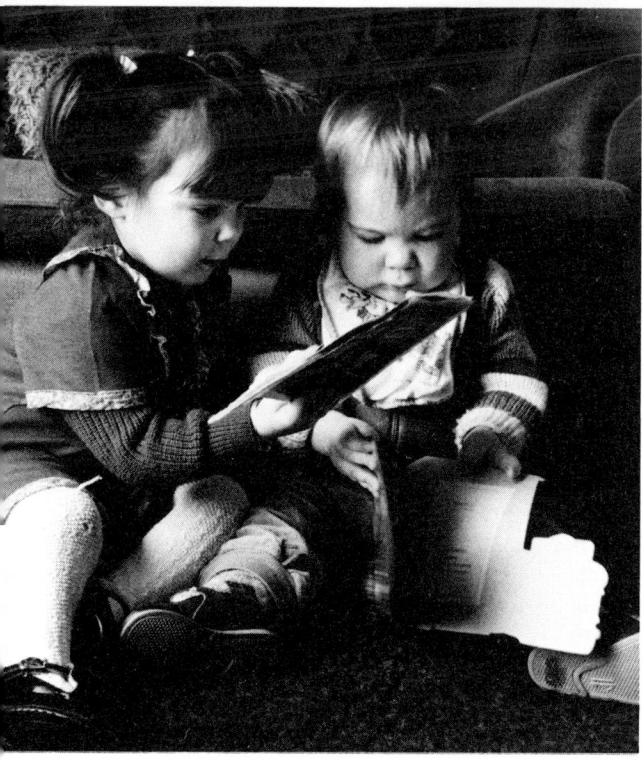
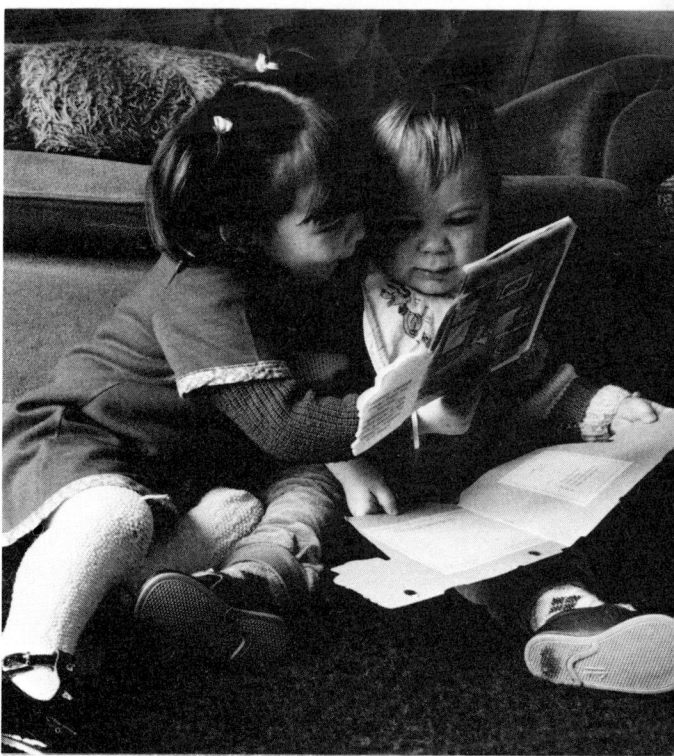

Talking to each other

We have already seen (in Chapter 6) how mothers alter their speech when they are talking to their babies and young children. They use short sentences; they repeat themselves; they ask a lot of questions; they 'feed back' to the baby the baby's own sounds and they interpret their meaning – even when, to anyone else, the baby's sounds do not seem to have any meaning!

It is natural for you, as a parent, to behave like this. You are deeply interested in your baby's development and keen to spot signs of progress and to build on them in a way that you feel will be helpful. What is remarkable about some studies of pre-school children talking to even younger children is that they, too, are able to modify their speech. One study of four-year-olds talking to two-year-olds found that the four-year-olds behaved very similarly to the mothers when talking to the two-year-olds.[55] They used shorter sentences than they did to other four-year-olds and adults; they asked a lot of questions and they repeated themselves helpfully. This indicates not only a very confident grasp of the different ways in which language can be used, but also the important quality mentioned above: the ability to see the other person's point of view. These young children *knew* that toddlers were not as linguistically knowledgeable as they themselves were – and they were able to produce the kinds of comments that they thought would be helpful in getting the little ones to understand.

It could be said that the four-year-olds were just imitating the adults when they altered their speech to the two-year-olds, and there is certainly an element of imitation in many utterances made by older to younger children: 'How many times have I told you not to touch the radiator?' But, in most aspects of speech and behaviour, four-year-olds have got way beyond the imitation stage; they are independent and creative people. Judy Dunn and Carol Kendrick found some interesting differences between the children and the mothers in their study of second babies and their families. A *very* high proportion of the comments made by the older to the younger child were orders: the older child was forever trying to stop, restrain or direct the younger child, frequently in play situations. In short, a second baby in a family seems to be subjected to a great deal of bossing around! The older children also went in for a lot of 'attention-getting' remarks: 'Hey.' 'Look.' 'Watch me.' 'You do it.' and so on. All this ordering about differed very much from the way the *mothers* talked to the younger children. A typical example of this is two-and-a-half-year-old Thomas to ten-month-old Hannah: 'Don't let Hannah have the play-dough. Don't go near the electric point, Hannah. Very dangerous. Be careful Hannah. Let Hannah have the sticklebricks.'

There are four instructions here. Three of them are prohibitions and one is a warning. 'Don't' and 'let' are repeated. It is also very striking that the older child is putting himself in the younger child's place. He knows that the electric point is dangerous for her and he knows that she does not know. He also knows that play-dough, while quite suitable for him to play with, is not suitable for her, because she might eat it.

It would be interesting to know the long-term effect of these constant instructions on the language development of younger children in the family – but, as yet, we lack the evidence. It might be good to reverse roles occasionally and give your older child the chance to be the younger one by finding an older friend for him to play with. Similarly, the second or later child may benefit by having to be the 'sensible', bossy older child to a younger playmate.

Twins

A twin (or triplet or quad) has a brother or sister as a companion from the beginning. The experience of twins in communicating with one another is going to be different from the experience of a pair in which one child is older and one younger. Twins are developing together although their individual rates of development may be different, with one twin taking the dominant 'older' role and the other allowing herself to be bossed about.

Even young babies can show an interest in each other's activities – as these young twins show.

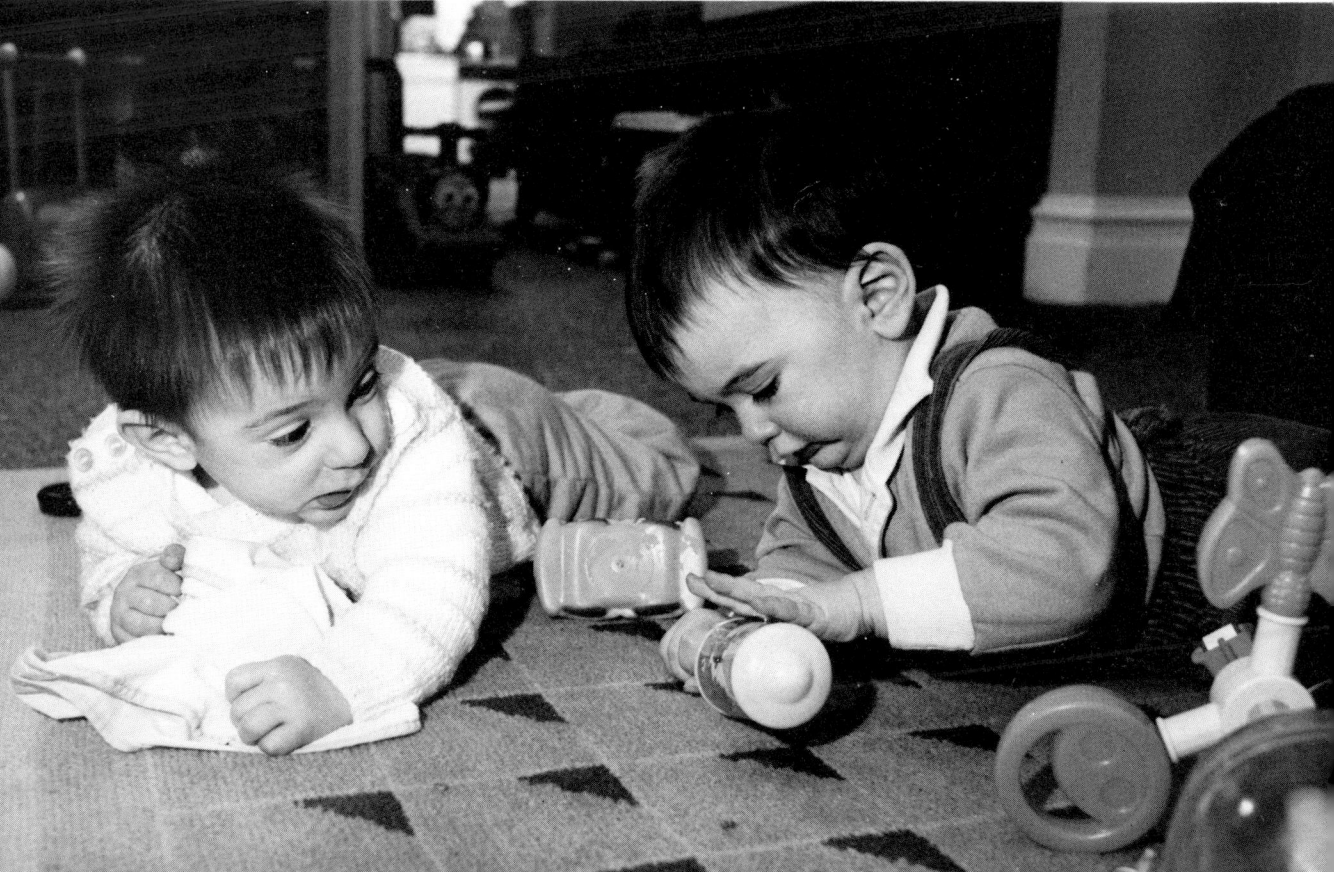

Twins can create special problems for parents in the everyday exchanges that promote the development of understanding and speech. Face-to-face contact with the mother during feeding or other caretaking activities generates the taking of turns and creates situations which mother and child can talk about. Occasions when the baby points or frowns or smiles or tugs at her mother's arm all contribute to the development of shared understanding and eventually expression in speech. But if there are two babies claiming the mother's attention, it will be very difficult and quite often impossible for her to give it to both. One baby will be attended to and the other's gestures and noises may be ignored.

Research on twins and their families has shown that, during feeding, the mother may be feeding one twin but actually talking to the other, especially if the other is getting rather impatient for her food.[56] The opportunities for 'conversation' during feeding are thus curtailed. It can also be puzzling for the baby who is being fed to hear her mother talking and to see her mother's expression when the voice and expressions seem to have nothing to do with what is going on (namely feeding), because the mother is talking to somebody else.

Twins may be left to each other's company a great deal, and they often get on well together and amuse each other. This gives their hard-pressed mother some breathing space. But it does mean that each child is more likely to hear her twin's attempts at language (which will be as immature as her own) than to hear the helpful adult. Twins and children of the same age generally cannot make the adjustments of their speech, cannot answer and ask questions, interpret, feed back and build on each other's attempts at communication as adults and older children can. This can mean that the twins do not get a clear model of appropriate language use, as described in Chapter 7, when the adult sees the child pointing to a pencil and saying 'nana' and the mother elaborates, 'Yes, that pencil is just like a banana.' The other twin may simply repeat 'nana' – and both the explanation and the opportunity to continue the conversation are lost.

Twins may also build up their own private world even more than other siblings do; they may take less notice of other people and be less likely to learn the normal rules and give-and-take of polite conversation. They may even develop their own words for things (as, indeed, do single children) which they share to the exclusion of other people although full private languages are much rarer than is sometimes thought.

All this sounds rather negative and depressing and there is some evidence that twins' speech development is slower than that of single-born children. However, none of it is irrevocable.

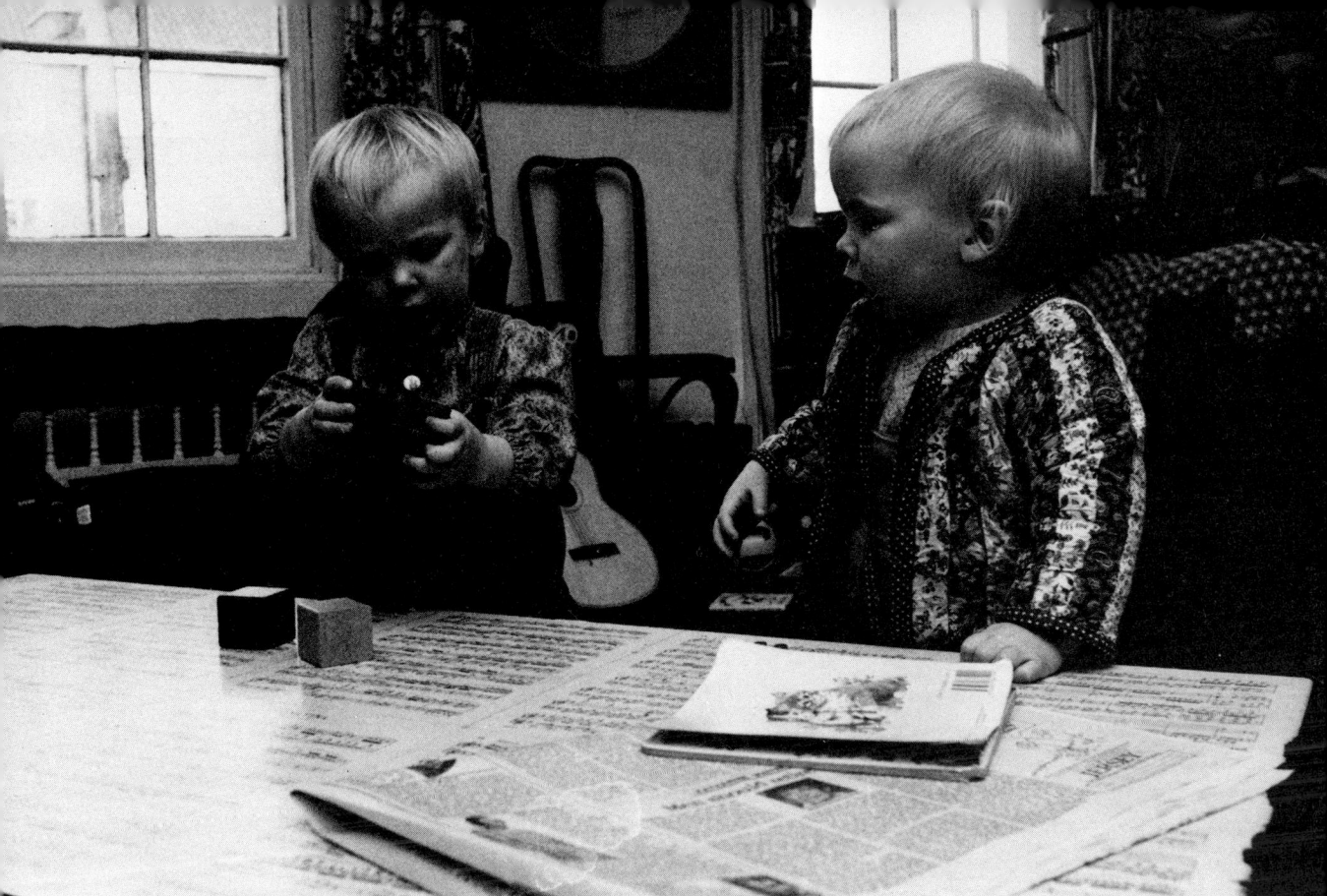

With a twin, you've always got someone to consult and to discuss things with.

You know the importance of adult attention in fostering understanding and conversation; it really is worth making time to give each child some individual conversation and play. It is also important to enlist the help of others – father, grandparents and older children, if you can find some. As they get older, twins will benefit more and more from the general advantages of having a brother or sister already described – co-operation (or, indeed, competition) in play and other activities, seeing another's point of view, and developing a quick understanding of the other's meanings. Some research has shown that twins can be so in tune with each other's speech that they can actually complete each other's sentences.[57] All this can be a great advantage, as long as you encourage them to share these skills with you and with other people. There is also evidence that, even where their language development is delayed, twins can catch up when they are at school. Good pre-school experience, where each child is encouraged to act as an individual, is even more valuable for twins than it is for other children.

Friends

Many people would find it difficult to accept that children who cannot yet talk in sentences can have 'friends'. It is true that young children who spend most of their time with their families do not have the opportunity to meet other children and this is the case with the majority of under-threes in the UK. It is also true that the sort of freedom to choose, to share interests, to make up games and join in activities together that older children (and adults) show, cannot be fully developed in babies and toddlers. Nevertheless, there is evidence to show that, when they are given the chance, babies and toddlers can display the kinds of skills towards each other referred to earlier in discussing babies' relationships with their parents and older children. These communication skills seem to be important in the development and effective use of language proper.

For example, research has shown that babies as young as three months will respond to other babies' crying.[58] They will turn towards the other child and perhaps cry themselves. This is something you may have noticed with your own baby. Even in the maternity ward, babies can set each other crying. When you take your baby to the clinic, you may notice that she becomes more alert, tries to look around and may imitate the sounds when she hears other babies crying or babbling. On these occasions, do give her the chance to observe and respond to other babies. You may be surprised at how much she enjoys it and how much social skill she shows, even when she is only a few months old.

Some researchers have deliberately put babies together to see how they would react to each other.[59] After six months, babies can definitely react to each other but usually for only one or two exchanges. These exchanges might be babbling to each other, or offering and taking a toy, or touching each other's faces and bodies or smiling at each other. The younger babies can quickly lose interest but as they get older the number of exchanges between them increases so that by a year one baby, for example, might crawl towards another baby and chatter at her, the other baby will turn to look and perhaps chatter back, then offer a toy which the first baby takes and examines and then will experimentally hit the second one with it. The second one cries, the first one reacts with distress and probably both babies will seek their mothers for comfort. This is quite a long sequence of exchanges and you can see that it is the foundation for the much more complicated play and conversations that three-year-olds can engage in: 'Can I play with you?' 'All right – you be the daddy and I'm the mummy.' 'Is this doll the baby?' 'No, that's not the baby.' 'Why not?' 'Because this one is.' – and so on.

Babies under a year can also show differences in how sociable or unsociable they are. One study of a group of eight- to ten-month-olds in a nursery found that there was definitely a most popular baby in the group.[60] The other babies more often approached her than anyone else and this was because she was more responsive, friendly and unaggressive. Similarly one of the babies was particularly 'unpopular'. The other babies avoided him because he was not responsive and was more interested in himself than he was in his companions.

It would be difficult to prove that these social exchanges between babies definitely affected their later language skills – that babies who were more responsive and better at keeping an exchange going turned out to be better at grammar or reading or writing later on. But if we see language not just as proficiency with words but as an expression of the ability to communicate effectively with other people, then it seems reasonable to suggest that babies who develop good communication with other children will have a good start in communicating with people, both verbally and in other ways, as they grow up. It is also important to remember that enjoyable exchanges with 'friends' are valuable in their own right: even if they do not have long-term consequences that can be proved, they will make your baby's and your own life happier and more rewarding. So it is worth trying to give your baby the opportunity to meet other babies and older children through mother-and-toddler groups or clinics or simply informal gatherings in people's homes.

Toddlers, from fifteen to thirty months, or so, get better at keeping 'conversational' exchanges going. As they are acquired, words will be added. One word can generate quite a complicated series of events:

First child: 'Teddy.'
Second child: 'Teddy?'
First child (grabbing the teddy): 'Teddy!'
Second child (trying to grab it back): 'No. Mine teddy.'
(First child refuses to let go.)
Second child (running to mother and pointing at first child): 'Teddy!'
Mother (correctly interpreting): 'Oh dear. Has Michael taken your teddy?'

This also shows another characteristic of baby/toddler communication that makes it different from the communications they have with their parents: exchanges between young children are far more likely to concern toys or other interesting objects. They are also more likely to end in tears than exchanges with adults are. It is important, though, that you allow your young children to have these kinds of experiences, precisely because they *are* different from the sorts of conversations they will have with you.

Children need to learn how to get on with different kinds of people and to adjust their speech and behaviour accordingly. The two children described above have learned a lesson about the nature of 'mine' and, by implication, 'not yours'. They have also learned something about the injustice of life and the need to find ways of dealing with it (in this case, as in adult life too, by appealing to a higher power). Later on, after repeated experiences of this kind, plus increased verbal skill, they will learn that there are rules of play that everyone has to follow if life is to be comfortable. There are also verbal ways of sorting out a dispute which can be done by the children themselves, without appealing to an adult. For example:

First child: 'Can I have a look at your car?'
Second child: 'Why?'
First child: 'Because it's like my dad's.'
Second child: 'All right. But only for a minute.'
First child: 'OK.' (Takes and examines car.)
Second child (after an interval): 'You've got to give it back now.'
First child: 'It's not a minute yet.'
Second child: 'Yes it is. You said you'd give it back after a minute.'
First child: 'All right.' (Hands it over.)

These two children have made a deal and, despite a small quibble, they stick to it. The first child can appeal to the second child's sense of fairness and be reasonably confident that he will get a response. Once they reach playgroup age, many children, particularly if they have had the chance to meet and play with other children already, will be able to make and keep the 'rules' in this way. Now, unlike the pre-verbal stage, these rules can be formulated and re-negotiated in language – a much more effective way of conducting business and settling disputes than hitting your companion over the head with a doll!

Boys and girls

Boys and girls do show differences in verbal ability, in talking, reading and writing, as they grow up. The differences are usually in favour of girls (although, as with all such general differences, there are many individual exceptions). It would be interesting to know what the origin of these differences are, or whether they can be changed if boys and girls are brought up more 'equally'.

During the first two years, in the early stages of language development, you may find your daughter quicker and more responsive at picking up language skills. She may speak sooner and acquire more words more quickly than your son. This may be partly because girls, on average, get a better start in life, physically, than boys do. They are less likely to have birth problems, to be handicapped or ill. There is evidence that they can discriminate between sounds better and earlier than boys. There is also evidence that the hemispheres of the brain in girl children start developing their separate functions earlier than in boys. It is the left hemisphere that is primarily responsible for language skills.

Other research suggests that parents pick up on these subtle physical differences and reinforce them.[61] Boys tend to be more irritable and active from birth. As they get older they tend to be encouraged to play more active games, which do not involve being close to an adult. Girls, on average, tend to be less active and more responsive to their mothers' speech and behaviour. Girls end up enjoying activities that adults can help with, such as painting, writing, or glueing. If you go to a mother and toddler club or to a playgroup you may notice that, in general, the boys run around and do things in gangs more than the girls do. The children getting lots of first-hand attention from an adult, at a table or busy in the Wendy House, are much more likely to be girls.

This is a very controversial area, and you probably have your own very definite views about how you want to bring up your boys and girls. But if you are concerned with *language* and the communication with and sensitivity to others that verbal skills involve, you might find it instructive to consider how you handle your little boy. How often do you converse face to face with him? How often do you cuddle him on your lap while you talk, sing or tell or read a story? Do you nod, smile, imitate, gesture, feed back, expand what he says and generally respond to his sounds and signals in the ways that we have been describing? Or do you feel he ought to be running around, climbing, building, playing with cars, and generally being more 'independent' of you?

Most of us are unaware of how we handle our children; we react to them quite unselfconsciously. So there is no suggestion here that anyone *deliberately* discriminates against (or for) their baby sons and daughters. For most of us, child-rearing practice is a mixture of what we already believe, our own experience (which modifies what we believe) and the ways in which our babies behave from the start (which modifies both our beliefs and our experience). But language skills can be improved and refined, and they are also a great source of mutual pleasure between parent and child. Some boys may be missing out on these pleasures, so if you have a son, or sons, try talking and listening to them as you would if they were girls. This is especially important if you are worried about their language development. (Slow developers are discussed further in Chapter 10.)

Other adults

Much of the research on language acquisition in babies and young children has concentrated on what goes on between the baby and her mother and there often seems to be an implicit

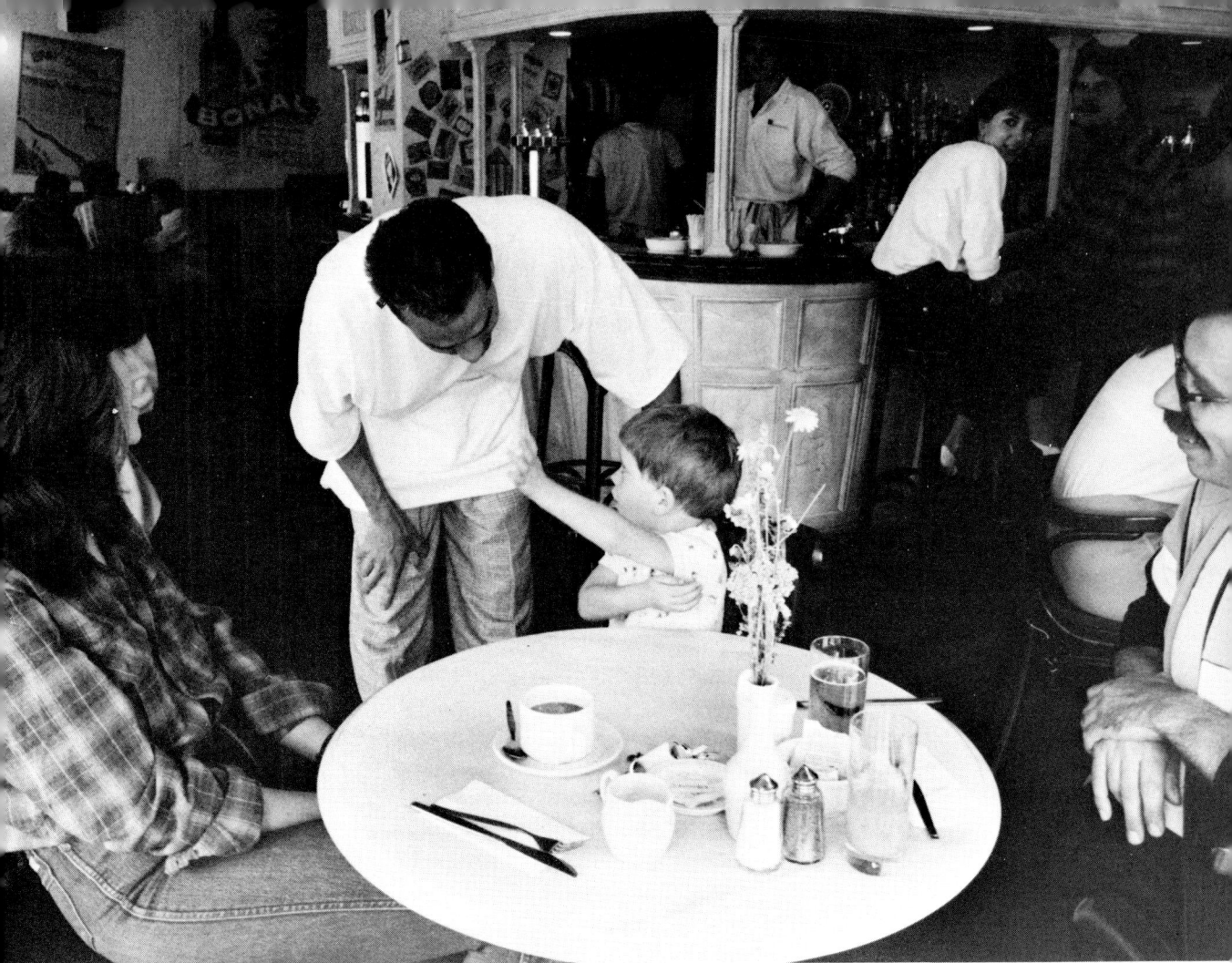

Children learn to get on with other adults, besides mum and dad.

assumption that it is *only* the mother who is having conversational exchanges with the baby. But, of course, this is not the case. Brothers and sisters can influence the picture. Babies also have fathers, who have been much less studied than mothers, but who have their own ways of relating to the baby, sometimes different, sometimes the same as the mother's. Many babies and toddlers have grandparents, aunties, uncles, cousins, neighbours, baby-sitters whom they regularly see. Every baby who is taken for a walk will encounter smiling shop-assistants, friendly elderly ladies, kindly postmen, milkmen and bus conductors. And, of course, many babies are regularly left in the care of other adults – either relatives, childminders or, more rarely in Britain, nursery nurses – while their mothers and fathers work, either part-time or full-time.

It should be obvious from what has been said so far that a lot of the caretaking and play that goes on between adult and baby right from birth provides opportunities for understanding, explanation and eventually spoken conversation. These kinds of exchanges are very intensive, with both adult and baby concentrating hard on whatever it is they are doing and on each other. They also rely on the building up of shared knowledge: the baby comes to learn, for example, that bathtime is a time for particular kinds of conversations. Special words will become associated with it: 'splash'; 'boat'; 'in'; 'out'; 'all wet'. Games such as 'This little piggy' while her feet and toes are being dried become part of the ritual and expand her understanding and eventually her vocabulary. Every family will have its special games, words and rituals for these occasions.

Thus, when a baby is left in the care of another adult, or adults, it is important for her language development (as well as other aspects of her life, such as her sense of security and emotional well-being) that these other adults provide similar experiences to those she would have in her own family: periods of intensive attention and sensitivity to her own ways of doing things – building up shared knowledge that both adult and baby understand. This means that she needs to be in an environment where she gets regular individual attention from familiar, affectionate adults. This can be provided by a good childminder or nanny or it can be provided in a good nursery. It cannot be provided by a childminder or nanny who has several (more than three) other babies and toddlers to look after or in a nursery where there are too few nurses to go round and where the care of the babies is rotated among different nurses all the time.

There is evidence that babies brought up in residential homes where they do not get much stimulation and where the care is rotated, lag behind in their language development.[62] It has also been found that when their system of care was changed, with more play and stimulation from individual nurses, their language skills improved. Similarly, babies left in poor childminding conditions, where the minder has a lot of young children to look after and does not know very much about their needs, may also be slow in understanding and talking. Such poor starts can be made up for, if the care is changed, but it is even better to avoid such poor care in the first place. When you choose a minder, nanny or nursery place, try to observe how the adults talk to and play with the children they are already looking after. Let the minder or nurse play with and handle your baby while you are there and watch how the baby responds. If you are happy with the way they relate to each other, and, very importantly, if *you* like the person, then you can feel confident about leaving your baby with her. If you are *not* happy, then look elsewhere.

One sign that your baby is not happy with substitute care is that she may go backwards in her language skills. She may be less responsive to what you say; she may babble and talk less; she may seem to 'forget' words and phrases she already knew. This can also happen after a spell in hospital. Such signals should be taken seriously; if possible her care should be changed. You can also make extra efforts yourself to provide happy times for play and communication and conversation at home. You may think that other 'professionals' know better than you do about how to stimulate your baby. Professionals certainly know a lot about babies in general, but when it comes to talking, it seems that home is best. A recent study of the language of nursery school children found that the language between mothers and children at home was richer than the conversations between children and teachers at school.[63] It covered more topics; developed lines of reasoning; used descriptions, memories of past events, plans for future events; discussed other people's feelings; explained how things worked. This was true of all social classes. Working-class mothers talked with their children just as fully as the middle-class mothers did.

Because we know that language skills are so important at school and for learning generally, we can feel that they are most appropriately 'taught' by 'experts'. Although it is good for young children to talk with other adults, *and* to attend school, the evidence seems to be that mothers, fathers and families excel above everybody else at encouraging the understanding of words and their confident expression in the early years.

9

Bilingual Babies

Hélène to her daughter, Renée (2½): 'Tu veux boire quelque chose?' Then, to Renée's English friend Sarah (2½): 'Would you like a drink?'

Hélène is French and married to Bill who is English. They and their daughter Renée live in London. Hélène feels no embarrassment in speaking French to her daughter at all times and translating what she says to Renée to Reneé's friends. Not all parents feel so comfortable operating in two languages. Sandra, also married to an Englishman, felt 'frankly anti-social' at speaking her native Dutch to her small daughter Lizzie in front of non-comprehending friends. This was such a problem for her that when her second daughter, Anna, came along, Dutch was used less and less in their household and her third child, Jeremy (eleven months), now only hears it when the family goes to Holland or is visited by Dutch friends and relations.

Which language? Making the decision

There are special problems involved in bringing up a child bilingual from birth in English and another language which is not spoken widely over here, such as the languages of the European Community. We focus here on this kind of bilingualism, not on that of speakers of the many minority languages used in Britain today. Languages such as Hindi, Bengali, Urdu, Gujerati and certain Caribbean dialects are often acquired as main languages before English is introduced after the age of three. The children learning them are usually able to communicate regularly with other members of the same language community outside the immediate family.

As far as the first kind of bilingualism is concerned, there are several things to consider once you and your partner have decided on a bilingual upbringing. Do you understand or even speak each other's language? In which country do you intend to settle permanently? Does the non-English speaking partner have frequent contacts with his or her speech community abroad?

You may want to bring up your baby bilingual in the 'classical' way, as Hélène and Bill have done with Renée: that is, with each parent using his and her own native language to the child, which has enabled Renée to become very adroit in switching from English to French and back. Or you may want to take a different approach because your personality or aptitude for language is different.

You may be surprised to find that your eventual decision, after the birth, is determined by your own emotions. You may find that babytalk only comes naturally to you in the language you were brought up in, even though you have been operating very efficiently in your adopted language at work for years. Pia, a Finnish girl, found that speaking her own language to her baby Daniel made her feel less lonely while her English husband, Ron, was at work. She had come to Britain as an adult and did not know the words and endearments used by English mothers to their babies. Babytalk in Finnish came much more easily to her. Because she was less confident in English than someone like Hélène, her baby Daniel did not benefit so much from the 'classical' bilingual situation, with father speaking one language and mother speaking the other. At two and a half, he spoke mainly Finnish.

Many mothers, though, feel reluctant to make the baby's father feel even more excluded than he might already feel after the birth of a baby. This was the case with Harriet and Tim when their daughter Edith arrived. Tim had acquired hardly a word of German, Harriet's native language, after six years of marriage. Edith was an early talker, speaking German to Harriet and to the German au pair and English to the father. In fact, whenever her father was present, she stubbornly refused to speak anything but English, which showed her ability to see her father's point of view, even at the early age of twenty months.

At twenty-two months, Edith could casually translate the main points of the conversation to an English visitor. Already, she was aware of the awkwardness of linguistic exclusion! Edith's mother Harriet had become completely used to speaking English at home and at work and eventually she and Tim decided to stick to English at home and to introduce German at a later stage. When their second child Ian was born, Harriet stopped using German so freely to Edith and now that Ian, a slow talker in English, is three, Harriet is teaching German to both children as a second language.

If you use your native language so infrequently that using it to your baby sounds stilted, you may prefer to stick to the language of the country you are living in.

In some situations, two languages may be needed.

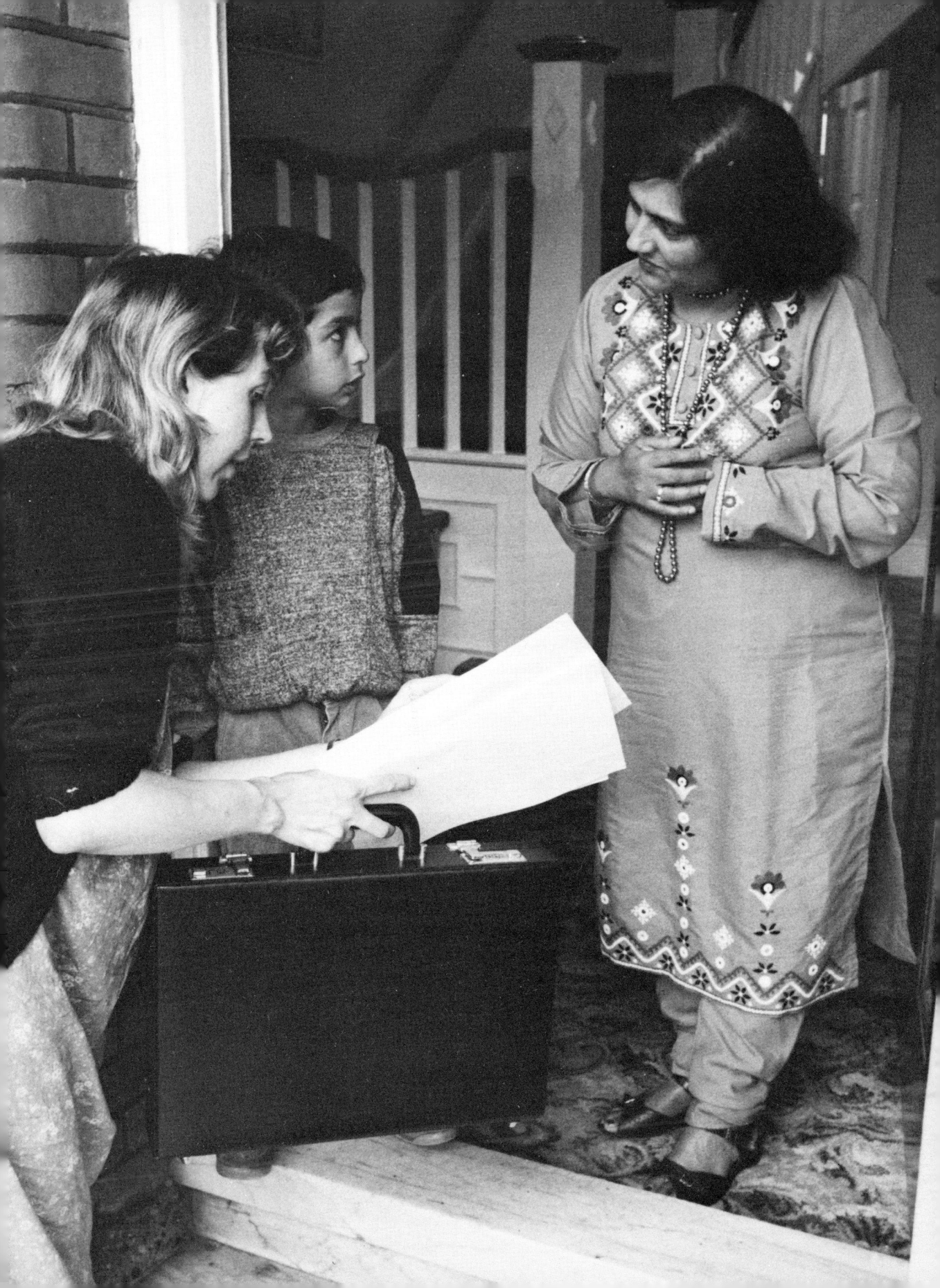

With a first baby, and whatever the circumstances, the decision at birth will be entirely up to you. Your baby will adjust to any situation you choose to present him with and will respond to whatever language you choose to talk to him in.[64] Not until the second year will *his* reactions and temperament begin to play a role. Then, he may influence you to review your earlier decisions. With second and later babies, the decision may be influenced by how you got on with your first child and how the older sibling chooses to talk to the baby.

As explained in Chapter 5, your young baby will have no problem in distinguishing speech sounds in the two languages he hears. His babbling will include speech sounds from both languages and towards the end of the first year, his 'jargon' will contain sound combinations resembling words in each language. To prevent him getting confused between the two, it is best not to switch from one language to the other when you are alone with him, but to stick to one.

Even if you are temporarily stuck for a word, try not to insert 'foreign' words or phrases into your speech, but to think of another word that will do. There are occasions when your baby *will* become aware of the existence of two languages in his home, especially as he becomes more sociable and aware of other people's differing characteristics, as recent research has shown.[65] When all three of you are together, you may switch to the other parent's language if he or she does not share yours. In the case of Pia and Ron, she would not speak Finnish to her son, Daniel, when Ron was around, but would use English to both of them. Similarly, your baby will come to recognise that one language only is used when outsiders are around.

Sometimes a child will use words from the other language to fill in gaps in his English, and vice-versa. Renée, fluent in French and English, sometimes says things like, 'Have a *cuiller*, Daddy', if she cannot for the moment remember the word 'spoon'. You can help your child to get things straight by giving him the correct word, saying: ' "cuiller" is French, in English it is called "spoon" ', and by making sure you are consistent in your own usage of words and grammatical rules. This kind of interference can worry parents, but there is good evidence that it passes quickly.[66]

'Interference' of this kind occasionally results in some delightful creative attempts at word-coining from young children. Anna (two and a half), looking for a word for 'pebble' in Dutch, came up with 'stonetje', a combination of the nearest English word she could think of plus the Dutch diminutive ending to indicate its small size.

Bilingual children in single-language families

The children mentioned so far all live in families which are bilingual, that is, where each parent has a different native language. But some children are brought up in families where both parents share the same language, but live in a different language community. When they settled in Britain four years ago, Ida and Hans, both Dutch, decided to bring up their children Michael and Eva (now six and four) as bilingual. At home, the family spoke Dutch and the children got their first real taste of English when they went to a playgroup at the age of two.

Michael, who was naturally quiet, appeared overwhelmed by the frustration of not being able to express himself and said not a word for a whole year. Eva, when her turn came, was better able to make her wishes known, reverting to gestures when her attempts to make herself understood failed. It took Eva and Michael more than two years to become fluent in English and their mother feels that, for them, each language is slightly different from the one language of most other children.

Recently Eva, who appeared to have coped so well, surprised her parents with a sudden outburst in which she bemoaned the fact that they could not always talk Dutch as they did when at grandma's. Although she is good at it, Eva seems to find the 'code switching' required at school a real effort.

Bilingual families who return to the country of origin of the parents discover that the second language is easily lost once the children start going to school there. On the whole, children become native speakers of the language of the country they live in, although they may well speak this language in a foreign accent for a while, as their parents do.

As the children improve their English accents, they may start to speak their parents' language with an English accent too. With some practice, bilingual children in single-language families can learn to speak both languages without an accent, just as children bilingual from birth can.

Children can be very irritated by the 'foreign' accent of their parents when speaking the language of the country they live in. When Carl (three) and Ronald (two) started playgroup and learned 'proper' English, they refused outright to speak English with their Swedish parents at home as they were embarrassed by their parents' slight foreign accent. Carl and Ronald's parents had wanted to help their children by getting in some practice at home, but this created another problem.

If the parents' English is poor, it can create a barrier between them and their children, once the children start mixing in the world outside. The children may not have the vocabulary at their disposal to describe their experiences outside adequately. Some-

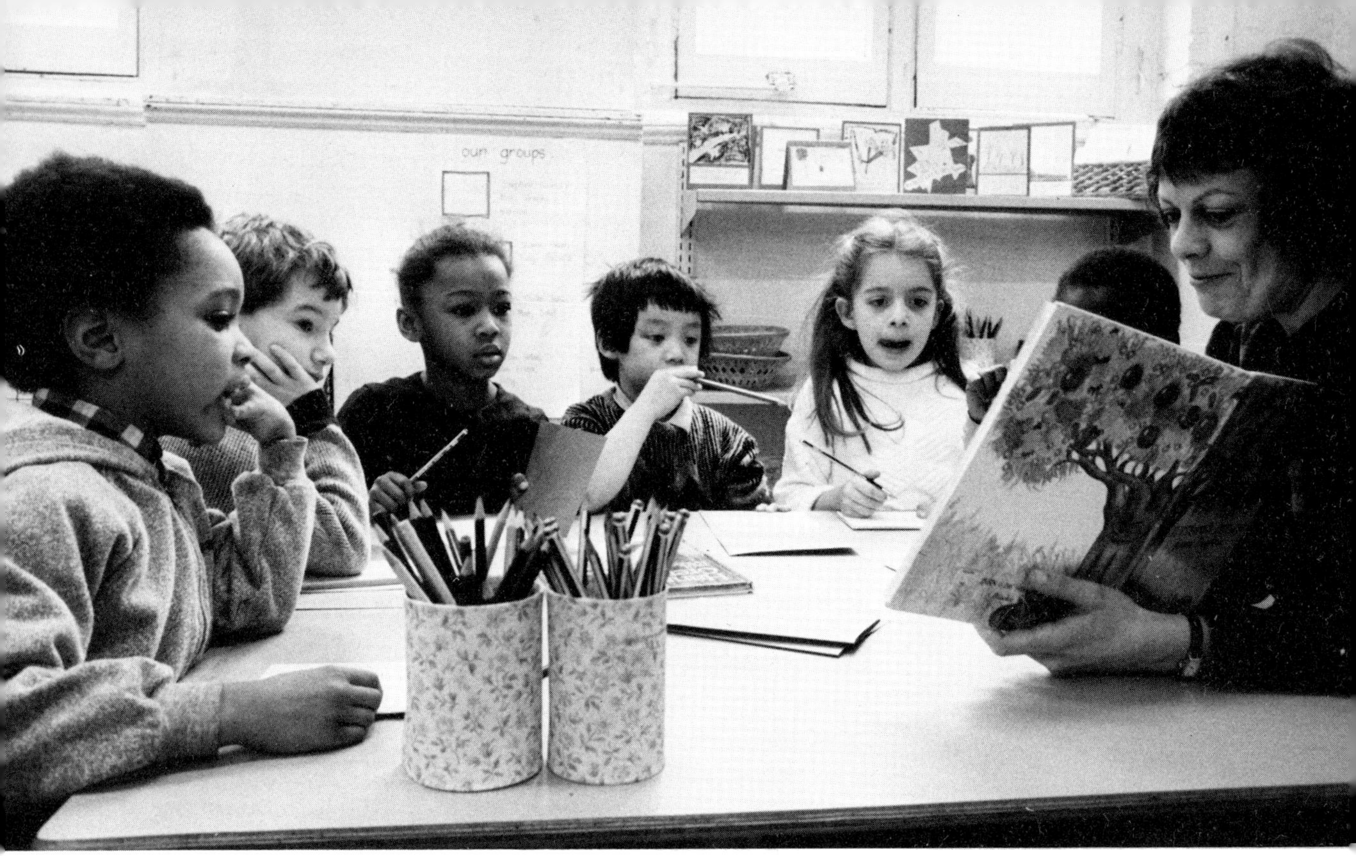

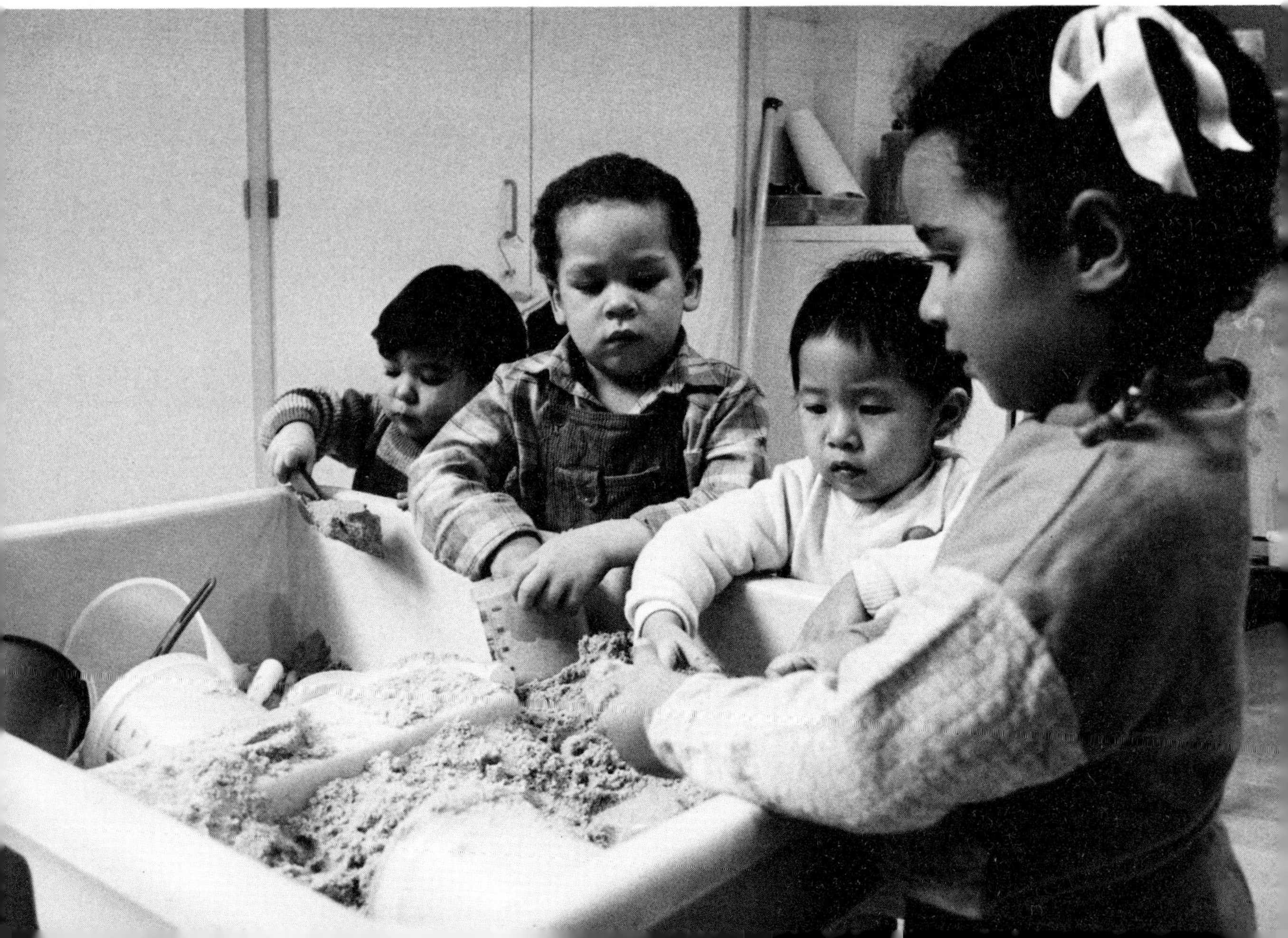

Children of different cultures and languages learn to communicate with each other in the school setting.

times, however, the children become expert interpreters, especially for mothers stuck at home and suffering the loneliness of not sharing the language of the community they live in. Local authority EFL (English as a Foreign Language) classes can fulfil an important function in helping family harmony.

Siblings and playmates

In Chapter 7, we discussed how even very young children can be influenced by other children. Not sharing the same language with his friends can be a social handicap for the bilingual child who hears a different language at home. Frustration at being misunderstood can lead to aggressive behaviour, not only in the non-English speaking children, but also in the English-speaking ones. Toddlers with calm and sociable temperaments seem to fare better at playgroups and in encounters with other children. Michael only started to speak English at his playgroup when it was joined by a Dutch helper who could act as his interpreter for a while.

Sometimes, though, sociable toddlers speaking different languages can form an instant rapport, even if one of them has no bilingual experience. The following conversation took place between three-and-a-half-year-old Kate on her first visit to the Dutch home of Ella, who was almost exactly the same age. Kate: 'Can I have the pram now?' Ella: 'Ja, dat mag.' (Yes, you can). Peaceful play continued with both girls chatting happily to each other in their respective languages.

Bilingual children may be less put out by communication difficulties than their single-language playmates, simply because they are more used to such difficulties and become quick at picking up useful phrases like 'Don't'. Their friends may not pick up a single word of the foreign language.

For bilingual toddlers growing up in single-language families it can be especially important to meet children who speak their 'home' language, so that they do not come to associate other children with problems in communication. Anna and Jake, bringing up their daughter Suzannah (two and a half) bilingual in English and Italian, have organised a network of Italian-speaking playmates for her who meet regularly at each other's homes. Suzannah also has English-speaking friends at the day nursery she attends. She shows the pride that many bilingual children can feel in their semi-foreign parentage by announcing pertly: 'I'm half-Italian!'

Experimenting with a bilingual upbringing is relatively easy with first or only children, but if there are siblings the pressures from the outside world become greater. The preferences of the older ones tend to have their effect on the speech of the younger

Play is a universal language for young children.

children. If the older ones happily switch to the home language, when back from school, or if they have no trouble speaking English to one parent and another language to the other, then the younger child will more often than not be happy to follow their example. But if the language of school is gradually becoming dominant in the older children, then the pressure on the younger ones to adopt the dominant language becomes considerable. Fortunately such younger siblings often develop an interest in the second language at a later age and still manage to become fluent in it.

Rather than insisting that the children relate their experiences outside to you in the home language, if your family is bilingual, you might choose to help them by allowing them to tell their playgroup or nursery stories in English and then supplying them with the relevant vocabulary in your own language. Edith, the girl who refused to speak German in her father's presence, would engage in protracted negotiations with her grandmother about where to speak German in the home. She might for instance consent to speaking German upstairs, but not downstairs on the one day, and the other way round on the next day. It is worthwhile trying to avoid the situation in which an attempted bilingual upbringing can turn the home into a battleground complete with linguistic zones, mirroring the political situation in certain bilingual countries such as Belgium or Canada!

Language and culture

If you are part of a large linguistic community in Britain, with its own religion, traditions, customs, rites and festivals, such as Hindu, Muslim, Orthodox Jewish or Chinese communities, it will be much easier to provide your child with rich linguistic experiences in the other language than if the other speakers of your language are scattered all over the country. If your children only have you as the person whose example they follow, and if your contacts with your own country are limited, their vocabulary will become a bit dated over the years. Of course, your children can update your language when they go abroad to visit friends and relatives, once you have given them a grounding in the basics.

Rich linguistic experiences consist in speaking and hearing a language in its cultural context, in knowing about the history, customs and beliefs of its speakers. It is a tall order for a parent to supply this experience in sufficient quantities to help the child maintain equivalence between the two languages he uses, if there is no language community to provide linguistic and cultural back-up.

Up to age three or so, it is not so difficult to match your children's English language experiences with similar experiences

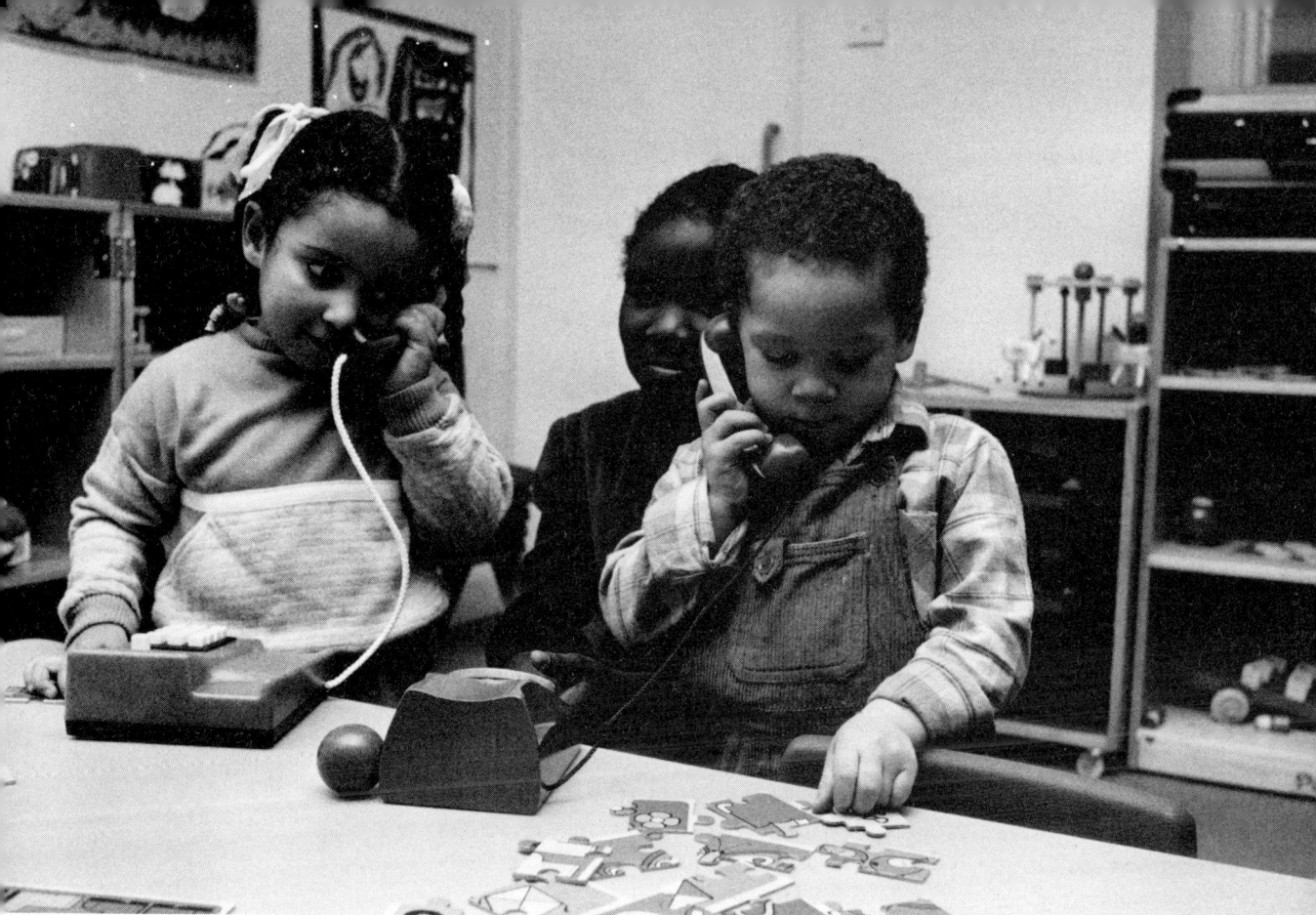

Children's easy acceptance of cultural differences.

in your own language. You can read them stories in your language, sing them songs and listen to children's programmes on foreign radio stations, if these exist in your language. Doing all this becomes harder when the children begin to spend more time away from you.

It is almost impossible to become equally familiar with the cultural traditions associated with the two languages you speak if you live permanently in one country. In bilingual families such as that of Sandra and Paul, regular decisions have to be made about the amount of emphasis to be given to different festivals. Will they celebrate Dutch 'Sinterklaas' early in December when Dutch children receive presents from a Father Christmas-like character? Or will they celebrate Christmas and receive their presents later in December? If Sinterklaas is dropped, their children will miss out on an essential experience of Dutch children, together with the vocabulary, songs and special edible treats that go with it. Accepting that celebrating both festivals is neither financially feasible nor educationally ideal, Sandra and Paul have struck a balance between them; they give their children token presents consisting of some typical Dutch sweets at Sinterklaas time. Children in larger foreign-language communities in Britain may not present such problems as children in isolated bilingual or single-language foreign families; these communities have their own festive traditions.

One of the advantages of growing up within a bilingual family can be the children's easy acceptance of cultural differences. 'Different' to them means just that; not peculiar or inferior as well. Between their parents there may be differences in such things as the way they hold their knife and fork, apart from personality differences. Noticing these differences can give rise to interesting discussions, such as why the law allows a cyclist to carry a passenger on the back in Holland but not in Britain!

Another advantage can be an early awareness of the phenomenon of language as a means of communication taking different forms in different people. Bilingual children become extremely sensitive to the linguistic abilities of other people and become aware of whether they speak both English and the foreign language, or only one of them. Kate, as we saw earlier, demonstrated this ability already in her second year. They often become intrigued by the possibilities of the two languages and want to know the equivalent word in the other language whenever they add a new word to their vocabulary. 'What's "cuiller" in English?' Renée will ask her father Bill. If they cannot understand someone, bilingual toddlers are quick to spot whether this is because the person is speaking an entirely different language or whether it is merely a gap in their own knowledge which is responsible for the misunderstanding. For the parents of bilingual children this linguistic perceptiveness is extremely interesting to watch.

Coping as parents

If you are trying to bring up your small children bilingual this will have a marked effect on your relationships with the other members of your community. For a start you will have to decide which language to speak in front of others to your child. If you are the 'other' speaker and hate the sound of your own voice in English, the choice will be relatively easy. Or, like Sandra, the advantage of being understood may outweigh the disadvantage of being embarrassed by your own voice. It may feel more comfortable for both you and your child if you agree to speak English in front of other children and adults, as when picking your child up from playgroup. You will be amazed at how well even very young children grasp 'social' rules like these. If you consistently speak English together in public your child is unlikely to take offence at any foreign accent you may have.

Always make sure that other adults your child meets know that a different language is spoken at home, so you do not find yourself in the position of Spanish parents whose three-year-old boy was put forward for speech therapy by a member of his nursery staff, because she had interpreted his thick accent when speaking English as a serious speech impediment.

Unsolicited advice will come your way, such as the frequently-heard observation that hearing two languages at home will delay your child's linguistic development. There is no good evidence that this is true. What evidence there is suggests that if your child is a keen communicator he is going to be a natural early talker in both languages, provided he is receiving equal exposure to them. Children who are by nature not terribly interested in using language early to communicate, who are perhaps solitary or at least not very sociable, may be reluctant to start using the two languages, but then such a child might have been a late talker even when only hearing one. Ian, Tim and Harriet's second child, said very little until he was almost two years old. When he was a baby they had already taken the decision not to use German as a daily language in the home, so English was the only language Ian heard. It was only around his third birthday that Ian started to be generally understood by people who were not closely involved with him and since then he has become extremely chatty. At the same time he began to be interested in the language his grandparents and his mother sometimes spoke and at age three and a half he now cheerfully experiments with the second language whenever he meets a native speaker of German.

Older children make their own rules and games, whatever the language barriers.

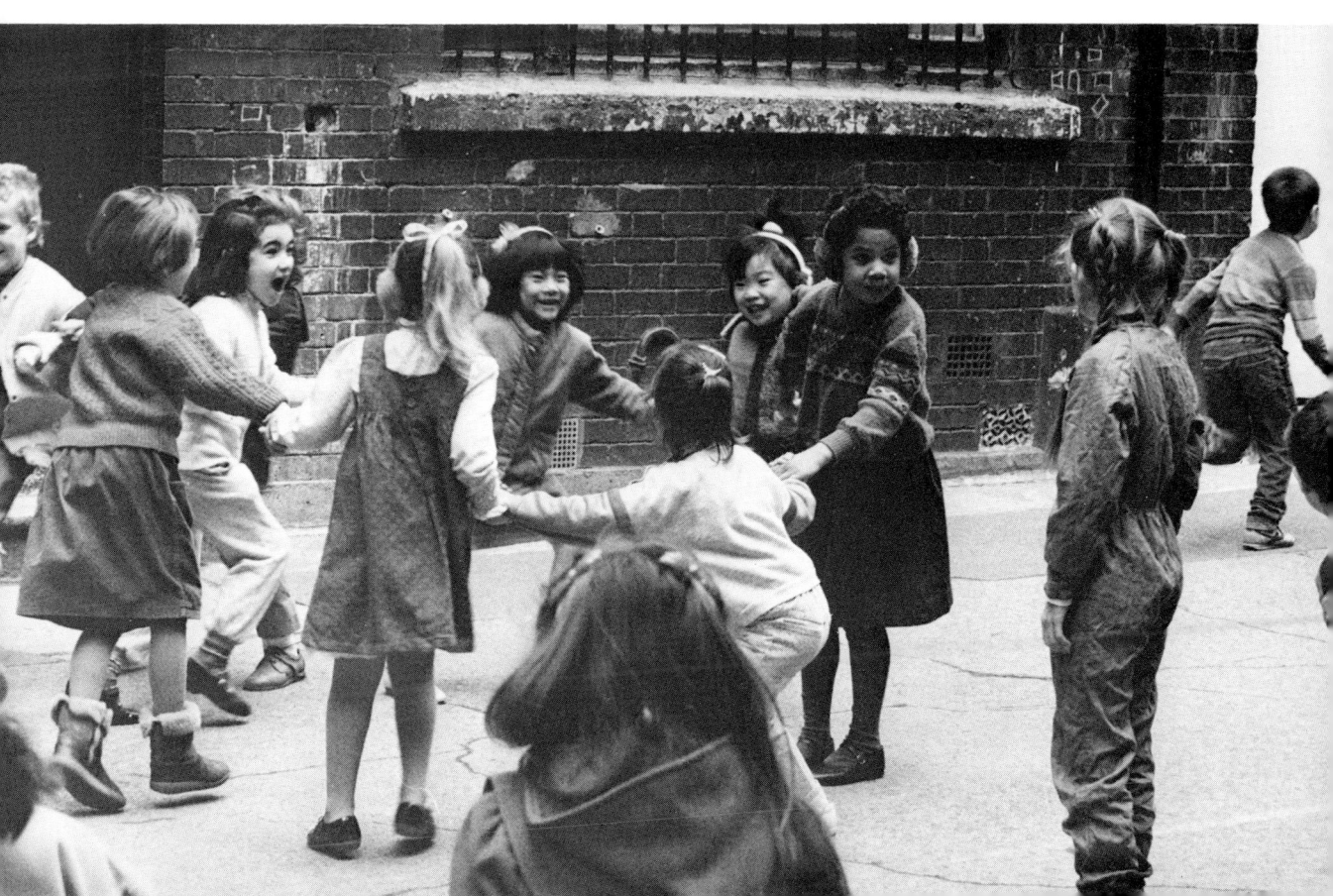

In the classical early bilingual development the two languages will be acquired at the same rate, with the restriction mentioned in Chapter 1, that the order in which certain grammatical constructions emerge in each language depends on their relative complexity.

If their bilingualism is to be an asset rather than a handicap you ought to bear in mind that your children need a considerable dose of 'cultural context' in both languages after the first few years.

If after a happy start you have begun to experience the consistent linguistic behaviour that is required of you as a bit of a strain and you are contemplating giving up on the bilingual experiment, you may feel reassured by the knowledge that however hard you practise with your children in the first few years, one language nevertheless tends to become dominant in the course of time. Usually, this is the main language of the country you live in. It is quite possible to supply your children with a near-native command of a second language if the second language is learned more deliberately at a slightly later age. Whether the outcome is bilingualism or semi-bilingualism you will have the satisfaction of giving your children the opportunity to speak a second language almost certainly better than they would have done otherwise. Quite probably you will have supplied them with a somewhat broader outlook on life, people and the differences between them.

10
Is Language Developing Normally?

Reasons for language problems
A constant idea throughout this book is that all your baby's skills and senses are potentially involved in the development of communication and language: hearing, sight, movement, touch, sociability. If any of these functions are damaged, either through congenital handicap, or through injury at birth, or through later injury or illness, this damage can hamper language development. Some forms of handicap are more disabling to language than others, deafness being the obvious example. If a child is mentally handicapped, for instance, a Downs' syndrome child, or is brain-damaged, *all* her intellectual abilities will be affected, including language skills.

Other forms of handicap, such as blindness or injuries which prevent her moving about, such as spina bifida, will not directly affect her hearing, verbal comprehension or speech – but they can make it more difficult for her to *understand* the world she lives in and to gain experiences from it, and thus make language learning harder for her. They can also influence the attitudes of other people, who may not know how to respond to her or to encourage the skills she has.

Some children may have no problem in understanding but have difficulty with the motor skills involved in articulating words: their *speech* will be affected. Examples are children born with cleft palates or children with cerebral palsy who cannot control the movements of their mouths and tongues. Some Downs' syndrome children may have this problem, too. Such problems can be greatly helped by skilled speech therapy.

If you have a child with one of these problems, the process of language acquisition will not be such a straightforward process as we described in Chapter 1. You have to work harder and give the child more conscious practice in listening, understanding and speaking. But many techniques exist for helping your child. The books and organisations listed at the end of the chapter, as well as your own doctors, health visitors and speech therapists, can all give you help and ideas – as can other parents with similar problems.

Recognising a problem

When a baby is born, she is tested to see whether her muscles, reflexes and perceptual responses are working properly. Can she see? Can she hear? Can she react? Can she move her head and limbs? Can she suck? It is possible to pick up some of the problems affecting language development at birth, or soon after – although some, such as the *extent* and type of a baby's hearing loss, may not become apparent until later.

Most babies 'pass' these early tests with no problems. But if there is cause for concern, they will be given further tests. Analysis of a baby's crying, using the kinds of techniques described in Chapter 3, can reveal abnormal patterns which could indicate brain damage. If you have reason to suspect hearing loss, for example, if you have deafness in the family, or if you have had rubella (German measles) during pregnancy, a newborn baby can be specially tested for hearing problems. But such hearing tests will not be done routinely.

Where a baby does not respond to light, or approaching objects, there will be cause to be concerned about her vision. Other major handicaps will be more immediately apparent – and help and treatment can start straight away. With language, as with other skills, the sooner a problem is identified and treatment begun, the better it is both for the baby and for you.

Can my baby hear?

How do you know if your baby has hearing problems? If she does not turn her head to sounds, or respond to your voice with smiles and limb movements, this is a possible sign. If she looks surprised to see you when you appear over her crib or cot, this may mean she has not heard the door open or your footsteps approaching. The baby with hearing loss will find many of the things she sees startling, as she will have had no warning from their sound that they were there.

Deaf babies do cry, gurgle and start to babble at the same age as other babies do, but this babbling will not develop into jargon and recognisable single words, as hearing babies' noises do. Eventually the deaf baby falls silent. All babies in the UK have a routine hearing test at about six to seven months which should pick up hearing problems. It is wise to ask for a test at any time you suspect your child's hearing is faulty. If she asks you to repeat everything; if she does not seem to understand what people say to her; if she mispronounces a lot of words over a period of

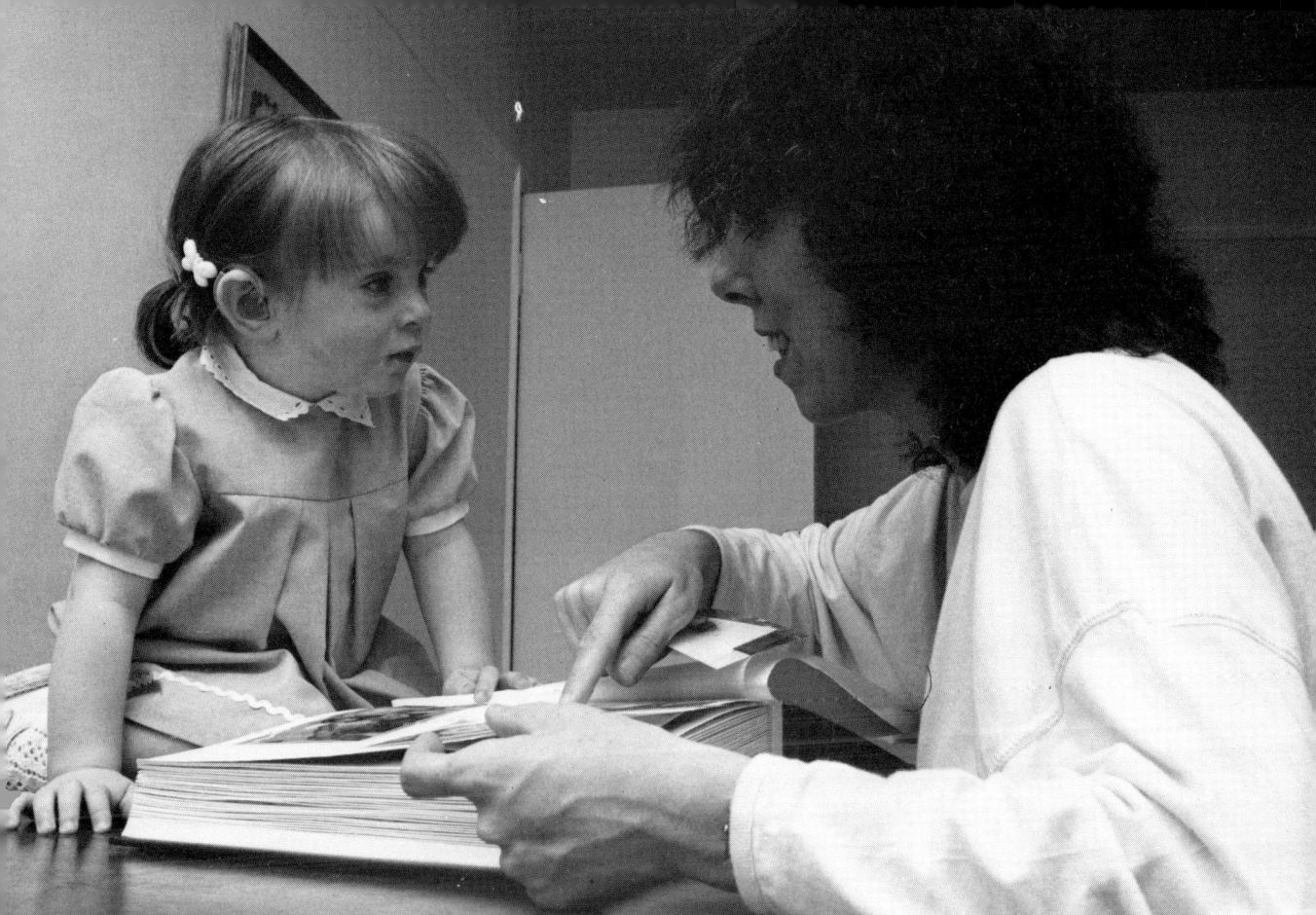

When a child can't hear properly, her eyes are very important. Watching her mother's lips helps her to understand; pictures help too.

months; if she does not seem to be developing speech at the usual rate – particularly if she is still not talking by age two; if she does not seem to be adding new words and grammatical rules to her existing speech. All these are good grounds for testing her hearing. You should also have her hearing checked if she suffers a lot from ear infections.

Can my child understand?

Throughout this book we have suggested ways in which you can tell whether your baby understands you and the world around her: does she recognise you and particular people? Does she smile, laugh, respond to being picked up, spoken to and played with? Does she reach, point, gesture, demand with loud babbles and 'nonsense'? Does she have likes and dislikes? Can she answer questions by her behaviour, such as turning round expectantly when you say, 'Is Nanny coming?' Does she know what different things are for? Does she drink from a cup, put a hat on her head, put teddy to sleep in his crib? You will have noticed all these and more examples of her growing understanding and ability to interpret her environment during her first twelve to eighteen months.

The subject matter of this book ends just as your baby is beginning to join words together to make sentences, that is around her second birthday – although some children will be talking in sentences before that and some may take a bit longer. The check list below will give you some idea of whether her *understanding* of language at around two to two and a half is what it should be. Remember that individuals vary widely and these are only guidelines. But if you are worried that she does not seem to understand what you say or do, then do seek help. Language learning can overcome very adverse conditions and, with the appropriate help and advice, there are many things you can do to improve your child's comprehension and speech.

What can she understand?

Can she find things if you name them? If you say, 'Where's the doll?' 'Where's the door?' 'Can you give me the shoes?' 'Show me the flowers', can she point to them, or pick them up? Obviously, she will only be able to identify familiar items with ease, although you may be surprised at the extent of her knowledge. If you ask her, for instance, where the newspaper or the lawnmower is, you may find that she does know what these things are. She should also recognise pictures of such objects.

Can she point to several different parts of her body? This can be quite an amusing bathtime game, when bits of her are under the water: 'Where's your toes?' 'Where's your tummy?' 'Can you wash your ears for me?' 'Don't forget your neck...' and so on.

Can she perform actions if you ask her to? You probably ask her to do all sorts of things in the course of everyday living: 'Give mummy the plate'; 'Show me your sore knee'; 'Let's take your socks off', and so on. But you may be surprised that she knows how to tell the difference between 'in', 'on' and 'under'. You can play a lot of games using these concepts: 'Let's put teddy on the chair'; 'Can you put the bricks in the box?' 'Shall we look for the ball under the table?' Physical play with swings, somersaults or just being tossed up in the air can teach concepts like 'up', 'down', 'around', 'upside down'. All these should be familiar to your two-year-old, and you can encourage her to do the same kinds of things with her toys, to reinforce her understanding. She should also be able to recognise similar actions in pictures: 'What are these people doing?' 'Show me where the little boy has fallen over in the snow...'

Can she listen with interest to stories, songs, TV programmes, radio and give you some indication that she knows what they were about? Even if she cannot talk very fluently, you can get an idea of her understanding by talking to her about the story and noticing if she imitates the actions in it.

Can she pass a message on? She may not do it word for word, but if she can tell mummy that auntie has arrived or tell daddy that big brother wants a biscuit (younger siblings are often used as messengers in this unscrupulous way!), if only by gesture, this is a good sign of her understanding.

Does she have an idea of big, small, one, lots? Again, these concepts come up in everyday activities. You can ask her to choose the big cornflakes packet from the supermarket shelf, not the small one and so on.

Does she play with other children? By around two many children can co-operate with each other in games or imaginative play – and they can certainly communicate (as described in Chapter 8). If your child can understand another child and make herself understood to the other child, this can be an even better test of her comprehension than some of her activities with you. It is harder work getting your ideas across to a person who is not making a big effort to encourage and understand you as an adult does.

If your child can do most of these things, even if she is not saying very much, you can be reassured that her linguistic skills are developing normally. Ideas for encouraging more 'output' in the form of speech are given in the next section. But if she cannot understand many of these concepts and tasks by around two, then you might find specialist advice helpful. In the first place, her hearing should be checked.

If her hearing is all right and she is developing normally in other ways – walking, using her hands, relating to other people and so on – then she may have a specific problem with language. The first person to talk to is your Health Visitor and also your GP. They can refer you for further tests to a developmental paediatrician and a specialist in language and speech difficulties, such as a speech therapist. Your child will be tested using rather similar guidelines to the ones described above and you will be given helpful advice about how to encourage her understanding and language skills at home. Many, many opportunities arise for helping your child to improve her understanding and vocabulary in the normal course of everyday life, so your role and the role of other family members is vital. There will be no need for alarm at this stage. Your child may simply be a bit slower than others and may well blossom out at a later age.

Is my child speaking normally?

If your child is not speaking at all by her second birthday, you should certainly ask your doctor for her hearing and other language skills to be tested. A general check-up on her all-round development will also be advisable, to make sure there is no physical or emotional problem that is interfering with her progress; sometimes illness, a spell in hospital, emotional upsets such as separation from a parent can delay a child's development and speech.

By two to two and a half, your child's speech should be developing along the following lines:

A rapid increase in vocabulary from around 50–75 words to about 200–400 words should take place in the first few months of her third year. (Again, some children will have had this spurt sooner than two, others a bit later.)

Vocabulary now includes not only nouns and a few all-purpose verbs but words which enable her to extend her grammatical skills: prepositions such as 'in', 'on', 'out', 'up', and so on; 'wh' question words, such as 'what', 'when', 'why', and so on; pronouns such as 'I', 'me', 'you', 'it'. All these enable her to extend the length of her sentences and to extend the range of her expression considerably. She can now ask questions in order to get answers. She can refer to something by its pronoun, not just by its name – which means that she realises that *you* know what she is talking about when she says 'it' or 'she'.

Other grammatical skills will develop: plurals, possessives (dollies, dolly's) and an understanding of the difference between them. She can also issue orders – 'You do it' – and may be adding 'ing' to the ends of verbs. When you ask her: 'What's this knife for?' 'For cutting,' she may reply.

She will become more creative now; she will start the conversation more, instead of waiting for you. She may tell you what has happened to her, or what she saw on television, or what another child did.

Her memory will have improved. She can repeat longer sentences and may have learned some rhymes or TV commercials. She can imitate what other people say quite well.

She may have coined some words of her own; Thomas, at two, had a whole private vocabulary of his own – 'paint-tain' was the safety gate, 'tropes' were the rubber suckers on his bath toy, 'truckles' were the plastic lids on beakers of coffee bought in cafés. These were all items whose names were not part of familiar everyday conversation, so he devised his own names for them.

Mispronunciations are common at two, with special problems over 's' (often 'th'), 'r' (often 'w'), 'th' (often 'f'), 'l' and 't'. Consonants get muddled up, for example 'hostipal', 'loowy' (for 'woolly') and syllables get left out ('comfortal' for 'comfortable') – although the child will recognise if you say it wrong. So long as you can understand most of what she says, and her 'mistakes' are consistent, you need not worry about this. But if her speech is really unintelligible to all but the most devoted listeners and this

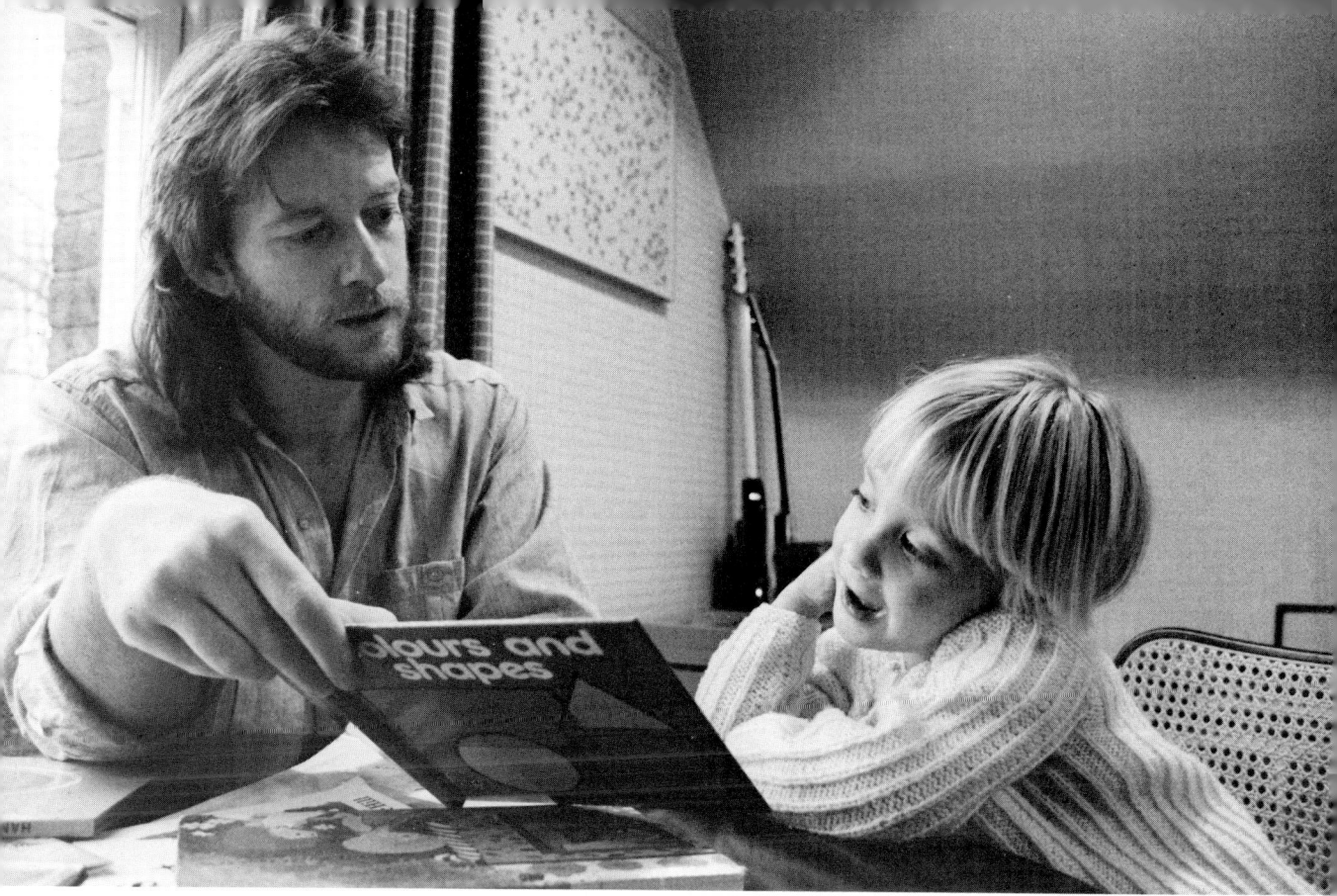

By two and a half, a child can be at home in the grown-up world of written language, with loving guidance from the people who've helped her to learn her spoken language. Words aren't just labels and commands any more – they're an entry into other people's thoughts, and the world of the imagination.

goes on until she is three, then you should seek advice and testing. Rhymes and songs which give practice in particular sounds, such as tongue-twisters ('Peter Piper picked...') and games which involve noises such as 'Shhhh' for the wind, or animal sounds ('moo', 'miaow') or 'boom, boom' for drums, can all help your child practise her articulation. You will be given more specific advice by your speech therapist. Play with other children and attendance at a good playgroup or nursery school, where the teachers understand the problem, can all help your child's powers of expression and her confidence.

Children who speak in a regional accent and use dialect phrases are *not* speaking incorrectly, even if their usages do not conform to the standard BBC voice. Fortunately, ideas about 'correct' and 'incorrect' speech are much more tolerant now than they used to be. It is important to remember that from a *linguistic* point of view, any form of speech which has its own consistent rules and grammar shared by a large community of people who all understand each other, is correct. So do not discourage your children from speaking in the tones and phrases that come most naturally to them; fluency, creativity and confidence are far more important in the development of language skills than the imitation of a 'foreign' (to them) dialect. Fluency and creativity can be hampered by forcing a child to speak in a way that does not come naturally to her. Interestingly, they can also be hampered by not allowing her to develop her own 'handedness' – the preferred use of right or left hand.

In her third and fourth year, your child will acquire nearly all of the main grammatical rules of her language and will be able to understand and speak to any other member of her language community, depending of course on how shy or sociable she is. But this is only the very beginning of what she can potentially do with her language. Language is not only utilitarian – a means of getting other people to understand what we want and getting it done. It is also the source of some of the most important pleasures in life. Conversation is one of the most enjoyable occupations in all communities of the world. Stories, rhymes, songs, poems all provide entertainment, and loving contact between parents and children and between children and their friends.

Later, reading introduces children to the ideas and experiences of people who have died or live in remote corners of the world, as well as of people like themselves in their own communities. Writing enables them to express and share their own ideas and feelings, as well as what they know. The complex linguistic worlds of newspapers, parliamentary debates, scientific discussion, theatre, cinema, commerce and literature still lie a long way ahead, but even when your child is a baby, she can start to appreciate the pleasures and possibilities of language through books, stories, conversations and games. Ideas for these activities can be found from some of the publications and organisations given in the Booklist and in Useful Addresses.

Useful Addresses

AFASIC (Association for all Speech Impaired Children)
Room 14, Toynbee Hall
28 Commercial Street, London E1 6LS

Downs Babies Association
Quinborne Community Centre
Ridgeacre Road, Birmingham B33 2TW

The College of Speech Therapists
47 St John's Wood High Street
London NW8 7NJ

The National Deaf Children's Society
31 Gloucester Place, London W1H 4EA

The National Society for Autistic Children
1A Golders Green Road, London NW11 8EA

The Spastics Society
12 Park Crescent, London W1N 4EQ

National Society for Mentally Handicapped Children
Pembridge Hall
17 Pembridge Square, London W2

Useful organisations generally

Books for Your Children
PO Box 507
Harborne, Birmingham B17 8PJ

The Federation of Children's Book Groups, c/o Books for Your Children

Cry-sis!
63 Putney Road, Enfield, Middlesex, EN3 G99

The National Association for the Welfare of Children in Hospital (NAWCH)
7 Exton Street, London SE1

The National Childbirth Trust
9 Queensborough Terrace, London W2 3TB

The Pre-School Playgroups Association
Alford House, Aveline Street, London SE11 5DH

All produce useful leaflets and booklets for parents, as well as being able to put you in touch with local groups.

Booklist

Baby and Child Penelope Leach, Penguin, 1983
Baby Gymnastics Arthur Balaskas and Peter Walker, Unwin Paperbacks, 1984
Babyhood Penelope Leach, Penguin, 1975
Book of Child Care Hugh Jolly, Allen and Unwin, 1985
The Bilingual Experience Eveline de Jong, Cambridge University Press, 1985
The Breastfeeding Book Máire Messenger Davies, Century, 1986
Brothers and Sisters Judy Dunn, Fontana/Open Books, 1984
Children's Talk Catherine Garvey, Fontana/Open Books, 1984
Crying Leaflet published by The National Childbirth Trust
Distress and Comfort Judy Dunn, Fontana/Open Books, 1982
Early Language Peter and Jill de Villiers, Fontana/Open Books, 1979
Encouraging Language Development Hastings and Hayes, Croom Helm, 1981
Fathering Ross D. Parke, Fontana/Open Books, 1981
The Growth of Sociability Rudolph Schaffer, Penguin, 1971
Infancy Martin Richards, Harper and Row, 1980
Let Me Speak Roy McConkey and Dorothy M. Jeffree, Souvenir Press (Condor Books imprint), 1976
Let's Help Our Children Talk Miriam Gallagher, O'Brien Press, Dublin, 1977
Life with Two Languages François Grosjean, Harvard University Press, 1982
Mothering Rudolph Schaffer, Fontana/Open Books, 1977
The Perceptual World of the Child Tom Bower, Fontana/Open Books, 1977 (reprinted in 1985)
Twins Averil Clegg and Anne Woollett, Century, 1983
Young Children Learning: Talking and Thinking at Home and at School B. Tizard and M. Hughes, Fontana/Open Books, 1984

Many picture and story books are now published for use with babies. 'Books for Your Children' (see Useful Addresses) can give advice, as can your local library. Babies can join the library in most places.

References

1 What is language?

1. H. L. Rheingold, 'The Development of Social Behaviour in the Human Infant'. *Monographs of the Society for Research in Child Development*, 31, 1966. Also K. A. Clarke-Stewart, 'Interactions between Mothers and their Young Children: Characteristics and Consequences.' *Monographs of the Society for Research in Child Development*, 38, 1973.
2. P. D. Eimas, 'Speech Perception in Early Infancy'. In L. B. Cohen and P. Salapatek (Eds.), *Infant Perception: from Sensation to Cognition* (Vol. 2). New York and London: Academic Press, 1975. Also P. D. Eimas, 'The Equivalence of Cues in the Perception of Speech by Infants.' *Infant Behavior and Development*, 8, 1985.
3. D. I. Slobin, 'Cognitive Prerequisites for the Development of Grammar'. In C. A. Ferguson and D. I. Slobin (Eds.), *Studies of Child Language Development*. New York: Holt, Rhinehart and Winston, 1973.
4. D. I. Slobin, 'Universals of Grammatical Development in Children.' In G. B. Flores d'Arcais and W. J. M. Levelt (Eds.), *Advances in Psycholinguistics*. New York: Elsevier, 1970.
5. M. K. Omar, *The Acquisition of Egyptian Arabic as a Native Language*. The Hague: Mouton Publishers, 1973.
6. D. I. Slobin, ibid., 1973
7. N. V. Smith, *The Acquisition of Phonology: a Case Study*. Cambridge: Cambridge University Press, 1973.
8. B. F. Skinner, *Verbal Behaviour*. New York: Appleton-Century-Crofts, 1957.
9. K. E. Nelson, G. Garskaddon and J. D. Bonvillian, 'Syntax Acquisition: Impact of Experimental Variation in Adult Verbal Interaction with the Child.' *Child Development*, 44, 1973.
10. N. Chomsky, 'Review of Skinner's Verbal Behavior.' *Language*, 35, 1959.
11. N. Chomsky, *Aspects of the Theory of Syntax*. Cambridge, Mass.: The M.I.T. Press, 1965. N. Chomsky, *Language and Mind*. New York: Harcourt Brace Jovanovich, 1968.
12. Herbert H. Clark and Eve V. Clark, *Psychology and Language*. New York: Harcourt Brace Jovanovich, 1977.
13. E. L. Newport, H. Gleitman and L. R. Gleitman, 'Mother I'd rather do it myself: some effects and non-effects of maternal speech style.' In C. Snow and C. Ferguson (Eds.), *Talking to Children*. Cambridge: Cambridge University Press 1977. Also L. R. Gleitman, E. L. Newport, H. Gleitman, 'The current status of the motherese hypothesis.' *Journal of Child Language*, 11, 1984.
14. R. F. Cromer, 'A Longitudinal Study of the Acquisition of Word Knowledge: Evidence against Gradual Learning.' *The British Journal of Developmental Psychology*, I, 1983.
15. P. A. de Villiers and J. G. de Villiers, *Early Language*. Glasgow: Fontana/Open Books, 1979.

2 What is a baby?

16. K. Kaye, 'Towards the origin of dialogue', in H. R. Schaffer (Ed.), *Studies in Mother Infant Interaction* (London, Academic Press, 1977).
17. J. Bruner, 'The beginnings of intellectual skill, 1', *New Behaviour*, 2nd October, 1975.
18. L. W. Sontag and R. F. Wallace, 'The movement response of the human foetus to sound stimuli', *Child Development*, 1935, 6. Also J. C. Grimwade *et al.*, 'Human foetal heart rate change and movement in response to vibratory stimuli', *American Journal of Obstetrics and Gynaecology*, 1971, 109, 86–90.
19. M. Wertheimer, 'Psychomotor co-ordination of auditory-visual space at birth', *Science*, 134, 1961.
20. E. R. Siqueland and L. P. Lipsitt, 'Conditioned head turning in human newborns,' *Journal of Experimental Child Psychology*, 3, 356–376, 1966.
21. T. G. R. Bower and J. G. Wishart, 'Development of auditory-manual co-ordination' in T. G. R. Bower, *Development in Infancy* (W. H. Freeman, San Francisco, 1974).
22. R. L. Fantz, 'Pattern vision in newborn infants', *Science*, 140, 296, 1963.
23. J. A. McFarlane, 'Olfactory factors in human attachment', paper presented at CIBA Foundation meeting on Parent Infant Attachment, London, Nov. 1974.
24. F. L. Fantz, 'Pattern discrimination and selective attention as determinants of perceptual development from birth', in J. Aline, J. Kidd, and J. L. Rivoire (Eds.), *Perceptual Development in Children* (University of London Press, 1966).

3 Crying

25. O. Wasz-Hockert, J. Lind, V. Vuorenski, T. Partanen and E. Valanné, *The Infant Cry* (London: Heinemann Medical Books, 1968).
26. F. Leboyer, *Birth without Violence* (London, Wildwood House, 1975).
27. J. Martin and J. Monk, *Infant Feeding, 1980* (London, OPCS, 1982).
28. A. McFarlane, *The Psychology of Childbirth* (Fontana, 1979).
29. M. H. Klaus and J. H. Kennell, *Maternal Infant Bonding* (St. Louis, Mosby, 1976).
31. J. Dunn, *Distress and Comfort* (Fontana/Open Books, 1982).
32. P. H. Wolff, 'The natural history of crying and other vocalisations in infancy,' in B. M. Foss (Ed.) *Determinants of Infant Behaviour 4* (London, Methuen, 1969).
33. S. M. Bell and M. D. S. Ainsworth, 'Attachment, exploration and separation illustrated by the behaviour of one year olds in a strange situation,' *Child Development*, 1970, 41, 49–67.
34. Y. Brackbill, 'Cumulative effects of continuous stimulation on arousal level in infants', *Child Development*, 1971, 42, 17–26.

4 Body language

35. R. L. Fantz, 'The origin of form perception', *Scientific American*, 1961, 204, 5.
36. A. N. Meltzoff and M. K. Moore, 'Facial and manual imitation by human neonates', *Science*, 1977, 198.
37. P. Wolff, 'Observations on the early development of smiling', in B. M. Foss (Ed.), *Determinants of Infant Behaviour II* (Tavistock Seminar on Mother Infant Interaction, Methuen, 1963).
38. W. Condon, 'Speech makes babies move' in R. Lewin (Ed.), *Child Alive* (London, Temple Smith, 1975).

5 Non-crying sounds

39. R. E. Stark, 'Prespeech Segmental Feature Development.' In P. Fletcher and M. Garman (Eds.), *Language Acquisition*. Cambridge: Cambridge University Press, 1979.
40. G. M. Haugen and R. W. McIntyre, 'Comparisons of vocal imitation, tactile stimulation, and food as reinforcers for infant vocalizations.' *Developmental Psychology*, 6, 1972.
41. E. Aronson and S. Rosenbloom, 'Space Perception in Early Infancy: Perception within a Common Auditory-Visual Space.' *Science*, 172, 1971.
42. D. K. Kuhl and A. N. Meltzoff, 'The Intermodal Representation of Speech in Infants.' *Infant Behavior and Development*, 7, 1984.
43. J. F. Werker and R. C. Tees, 'Cross-Language Speech Perception: Evidence for Perceptual Reorganization during the First Year of Life.' *Infant Behavior and Development*, 7, 1984.
44. C. M. Super and S. Harkness, 'The Development of Affect in Infancy and Early Childhood.' In D. A. Wagner and H. W. Stevenson (Eds.), *Cultural Perspectives on Child Development*. San Francisco: W. H. Freeman, 1982.
45. T. G. R. Bower, *A Primer of Infant Development*. San Francisco, W. H. Freeman, 1977.
46. E. Newport, 'Motherese: The Speech of Mothers to Young Children.' In N. J. Castellan, D. B. Pisoni and G. Potts (Eds.), *Cognitive Theory*, Vol. 2. Hillsdale, New York: Lawrence Erlbaum Associates, 1977.
47. K. Kaye, 'Towards the Origin of Dialogue.' In H. Schaffer (Ed.), *Studies in Mother-Infant Interaction*. New York: Academic Press, 1977.
48. C. E. Snow, 'The Development of Conversation between Mothers and Babies.' *Journal of Child Language*, 4, 1977.

6 The first words

49. D. I. Slobin, 'Universals of grammatical development in children', in G. B. Flores d'Arcais and W. J. M. Levelt (Eds.), *Advances in Psycholinguistics* (Amsterdam, North Holland Publishing, 1970).

50. K. Nelson, 'Structure and strategy in learning to talk', Monographs of the Society for Research in Child Development, 1973, 38, serial no 149.
51. K. Nelson, ibid.
52. E. Newport ibid. J. Jacobson *et al.*, 'Paralinguistic features of adult speech to infants and small children,' *Child Development* (1983), 54.

7 Two words and beyond

53. N. Katz, E. Baker and J. Macnamara, 'What's in a name? A study of how children learn common and proper names', *Child Development*, 1974, 65.

8 The wider world of language

54. J. Dunn and C. Kendrick, *Siblings: Love, Envy and Understanding* (London, Grant McIntyre, 1982).
55. M. Shatz and R. Gelman, 'The development of communication skills: modifications in the speech of young children as a function of the listener.' (Monographs of the Society for Research in Child Development, 1973, 38, no. 5.)
56. A. Clegg and A. Woollett, *Twins: from Conception to Five Years* (London, Century, 1983).
57. S. Savic, *How twins learn to talk: a study of the speech development of twins from one to three* (London, Academic Press, 1980).
58. M. Vincze, 'The social contacts of young children reared together' (*Early Child Development and Care*, 1971 (1).
59. M. Mandry and M. Nekula, 'Social relationships between children of the same age during the first two years of life' (*Journal of Genetic Psychology*, 1939, 54 (1).
60. L. Lee, 'Social encounters of infants. The beginnings of popularity' (paper presented at meeting of the International Society for the Study of Behavioural Development, Ann Arbor, Michigan, 1973).
61. C. Hutt, 'Sex role differentiation in social development' (in H. McGurk (Ed.) *Issues in Childhood Social Development*; London, Methuen, 1978).
62. M. Rutter, *Maternal Deprivation Reassessed* (London, Penguin, 1982).
63. B. Tizard and M. Hughes, *Young Children Learning, Talking and Thinking at Home and at School* (Fontana, 1984).

9 Bilingual babies

64. E. E. Garcia, 'Becoming Bilingual during Early Childhood.' *International Journal of Behavioural Development*, 6, 1983.
65. M. M. Vihman, 'Language Differentiation by the Bilingual Infant'. *Journal of Child Language*, 12, 1986.
66. K. J. Lindholm and A. M. Padilla, 'Language Mixing in Bilingual Children'. *Journal of Child Language*, 5, 1978. Also W. E. Redlinger and T. Park, 'Language Mixing in Young Bilinguals'. *Journal of Child Language*, 7, 1980.

Table 1 Stages of Development (from BOWER, 1974, p.185)

STAGE	AGE (in Months)*	SUCCESS	FAIL
1	0–2	No particular behaviour shown in response to hiding event.	
2	2–4	She will track a moving object that goes behind a screen. She can learn to track an object from place to place.	She continues to track a moving object after it has stopped. She will look for an object in its familiar place even when she sees object moving to new place.
3	4–6	She no longer makes tracking errors of Stage 2. She recovers an object which has been partially covered by a cloth.	She cannot recover an object which has been fully covered by a cloth.
4	6–12	She can now recover an object which has been completely hidden under a cloth.	She searches for an object in place where previously found, ignoring the place where seen hidden.
5	12–15	She no longer makes place error of Stage 4.	She cannot cope with invisible displacements of an object.
6	15–18	Complete success – she can find object no matter where or how hidden.	

* Ages are approximate; there may be considerable individual differences.

Index

anger crying 45
articles 88

babbling 9, 63-6
bilingualism 111-22
birth experience 24
boy and girl differences 106-7
brothers and sisters *see* siblings

childminders 108-9
cold 43, 49
communication codes 69
comprehension 80
constant crying 47
conversation
   babbling 64
   first year 67
   one-word 81-2
crying
   differences 38
   reasons 40-6
   soothing 48
   speech relationship 48
culture and language 118-20

discomfort 42-3
disputes 105-6
Downs' syndrome 123

eye
   contact 57
   movements 58

facial expressions 53-6
father's language 112
fear crying 44-5
friends 103-6
   bilingual 117
frustration crying 44

girl and boy differences 106-7
grammar 12
   constructions 16
   rules 14
   two-word 89-92

handicapped children 123
hearing disability 124
hunger crying 41-2

imitation 18-19

jargon 65

labels 13
language 11
   acquisition 19
   four-year old 14
   learning 15
   problems 123

manners 79-80
mispronunciations 78-9, 128
mother-language 69-72
movement
   communication 61-2
   control 59

negation 90
newborn
   eye control 28
   facial expressions 53
   first cry 38
   movement 27, 59
   perception 23
   sound perception 31
   sucking behaviour 28-31
normal speech 127-30

object permanence 34

pain 42
playmates 105
   bilingual 117
prenatal experience 23-4
problem recognition 124

regional accent 129
residential homes 109
rhythm 49

sensory perception 32
separation anxiety 69
siblings 94
   bilingual 117
   communication 100-1
   interpreters 95
   understanding 98
skin contact 43
smiling 56-7
sound
   perception 31
   soothing effect 49
stimulation 52
sucking
   behaviour 28-31
   enjoyment 49
swaddling 49

telegraphic speech 89
tone of voice 12, 80
translations 83
twins 101-3

understanding, development of
   20-1, 125-7

verb 'to be' 93
vocabulary 128

warmth 49
white noise 49
why?-questions 22

word
   combination 12
   endings 16
   invented 76
   order 85
   'sentences' 77
   single 73-4
   sounds 87
   topics 74